Rheumatol

T0229088

Editor

BENJAMIN J SMITH

PHYSICIAN ASSISTANT CLINICS

www.physicianassistant.theclinics.com

Consulting Editor
JAMES A. VAN RHEE

January 2021 • Volume 6 • Number 1

ELSEVIER

1600 John F. Kennedy Boulevard • Suite 1800 • Philadelphia, Pennsylvania, 19103-2899

http://www.theclinics.com

PHYSICIAN ASSISTANT CLINICS Volume 6, Number 1
January 2021 ISSN 2405-7991, ISBN-13: 978-0-323-75785-0

Editor: Katerina Heidhausen
Developmental Editor: Casey Potter

Physician Assistant Clinics (ISSN: 2405–7991) is published quarterly by Elsevier Inc., 360 Park Avenue South, New York, NY 10010-1710. Months of issue are January, April, July, and October. Periodicals postage paid at New York, NY and additional mailing offices. Subscription prices are $150.00 per year (US individuals), $290.00 (US institutions), $100.00 (US students), $150.00 (Canadian individuals), $297.00 (Canadian institutions), $100.00 (Canadian students), $150.00 (international individuals), $297.00 (international institutions), and $100.00 (international students). Foreign air speed delivery is included in all *Clinics* subscription prices. All prices are subject to change without notice. POSTMASTER: Send address changes to *Physician Assistant Clinics*, Elsevier Periodicals Customer Service, 11830 Westline Industrial Drive, St. Louis, MO 63146. Customer Service Health Sciences Division, Subscription Customer Service, 3251 Riverport Lane, Maryland Heights, MO 63043. **Customer Service: 1-800-654-2452 (U.S. and Canada); 314-447-8871 (outside U.S. and Canada). Fax: 314-447-8029. E-mail: journalscustomerservice-usa@elsevier.com (for print support); journalsonlinesupport-usa@elsevier.com (for online support).**

Reprints. For copies of 100 or more, of articles in this publication, please contact the Commercial Reprints Department, Elsevier Inc., 360 Park Avenue South, New York, NY 10010-1710. Tel. 212-633-3874; Fax: 212-633-3820; E-mail: reprints@elsevier.com.

Physician Assistant Clinics is covered in *EMBASE/Excerpta Medica and ESCI.*

PROGRAM OBJECTIVE
The goal of the *Physician Assistant Clinics* is to keep practicing physician assistants up to date with current clinical practice by providing timely articles reviewing the state of the art in patient care.

TARGET AUDIENCE
Physician Assistants and other healthcare professionals

LEARNING OBJECTIVES
Upon completion of this activity, participants will be able to:
1. Review the main components and function of the immune system and its role in rheumatic disease.
2. Discuss the classification and multisystemic manifestations of idiopathic inflammatory myopathies (IIM).
3. Recognize the impact of pediatric rheumatic disease including disturbed growth and development, negative psychosocial implications, altered family dynamics and risk of morbidities in adulthood.

ACCREDITATION
The Elsevier Office of Continuing Medical Education (EOCME) is accredited by the Accreditation Council for Continuing Medical Education (ACCME) to provide continuing medical education for physicians.

The EOCME designates this journal-based CME activity for a maximum of 14 *AMA PRA Category 1 Credit*(s)™. Physicians should claim only the credit commensurate with the extent of their participation in the activity.

All other healthcare professionals requesting continuing education credit for this enduring material will be issued a certificate of participation.

DISCLOSURE OF CONFLICTS OF INTEREST
The EOCME assesses conflict of interest with its instructors, faculty, planners, and other individuals who are in a position to control the content of CME activities. All relevant conflicts of interest that are identified are thoroughly vetted by EOCME for fair balance, scientific objectivity, and patient care recommendations. EOCME is committed to providing its learners with CME activities that promote improvements or quality in healthcare and not a specific proprietary business or a commercial interest.

The planning committee, staff, authors and editors listed below have identified no financial relationships or relationships to products or devices they or their spouse/life partner have with commercial interest related to the content of this CME activity:
Kirsten R. Ambrose, MS, CCRC; Heather Benham, DNP, APRN, CPNP-PC; Esther Bennitta; Leigh F. Callahan, PhD; Regina Chavous-Gibson, MSN, RN; Brigitta J. Cintron, DMSc, PA-C; Teresa M. Crout, MD, FACR; Kristin M. D'Silva, MD; Joan Doback, MHP, PA-C; Ariadne V. Ebel, DO; Michael G. Feely, MD; Katerina Heidhausen; Katie F. Huffman, MA; Anand Kumthekar, MBBS; Day S. Lennep, MD, FACP, FACR; Vikas Majithia, MD, MPH, FACP, FACR; Joan McTigue, PA-C, MS; Amanda E. Nelson, MD, MSCR; James R. O'Dell, MD, MACP, MACR; Richard Pope, MPAS, PA-C, DFAAPA, CPAAPA; Casey Potter; Carrie Schreibman, MSN, FNP; Barbara A. Slusher, MSW, PA-C; Benjamin J Smith, DMSc, PA-C, DFAAPA; Tina H. Thornhill, PharmD, FASCP, BCGP; James A. Van Rhee, MS, PA-C; Tracey B. Wright, MD

The planning committee, staff, authors and editors listed below have identified financial relationships or relationships to products or devices they or their spouse/life partner have with commercial interest related to the content of this CME activity:
Marcy B. Bolster, MD: research support from AbbVie Inc., Amgen Inc., Corbus Pharmaceuticals Holdings, Inc., Cumberland Pharmaceuticals Inc., Genentech, USA Inc., and Pfizer Inc.; owns stock in Johnson & Johnson Services, Inc.

Atul Deodhar, MD, FRCP: consultant/advisor for Amgen Inc, Boehringer Ingelheim International GmbH, Celgene Corporation, A Bristol-Myers Squibb Company, and Galapagos NV; consultant/advisor and research support from AbbVie Inc., Eli Lilly and Company, GlaxoSmithKline plc, Novartis AG, Pfizer Inc., and UCB, Inc.

UNAPPROVED/OFF-LABEL USE DISCLOSURE
The EOCME requires CME faculty to disclose to the participants:
1. When products or procedures being discussed are off-label, unlabelled, experimental, and/or investigational (not US Food and Drug Administration [FDA] approved); and

2. Any limitations on the information presented, such as data that are preliminary or that represent ongoing research, interim analyses, and/or unsupported opinions. Faculty may discuss information about pharmaceutical agents that is outside of FDA-approved labelling. This information is intended solely for CME and is not intended to promote off-label use of these medications. If you have any questions, contact the medical affairs department of the manufacturer for the most recent prescribing information.

TO ENROLL
The CME program is available to all *Physician Assistant Clinics* subscribers at no additional fee. To subscribe to the *Physician Assistant Clinics*, call customer service at 1-800-654-2452 or sign up online at www.physicianassistant.theclinics.com/.

METHOD OF PARTICIPATION
In order to claim credit, participants must complete the following:
1. Complete enrolment as indicated above
2. Read the activity
3. Complete the CME Test and Evaluation. Participants must achieve a score of 70% on the test. All CME Tests and Evaluations must be completed online

CME INQUIRIES/SPECIAL NEEDS
For all CME inquiries or special needs, please contact elsevierCME@elsevier.com.

Contributors

CONSULTING EDITOR

JAMES A. VAN RHEE, MS, PA-C
Associate Professor, Program Director, Yale School of Medicine, Yale Physician Assistant Online Program, New Haven, Connecticut

EDITOR

BENJAMIN J SMITH, DMSc, PA-C, DFAAPA
Director of Didactic Education, Assistant Professor, Florida State University College of Medicine, School of Physician Assistant Practice, Tallahassee, Florida; Rheumatology Physician Assistant, McIntosh Clinic, PC, Thomasville, Georgia

AUTHORS

KIRSTEN R. AMBROSE, MS, CCRC
Osteoarthritis Action Alliance, Thurston Arthritis Research Center, The University of North Carolina at Chapel Hill, Chapel Hill, North Carolina

HEATHER BENHAM, DNP, APRN, CPNP-PC
Pediatric Nurse Practitioner, Pediatric Rheumatology, Scottish Rite Hospital, Dallas, Texas

MARCY B. BOLSTER, MD
Associate Professor of Medicine, Division of Rheumatology, Allergy, and Immunology, Massachusetts General Hospital, Boston, Massachusetts

LEIGH F. CALLAHAN, PhD
Professor of Medicine, Osteoarthritis Action Alliance, Thurston Arthritis Research Center, Departments of Medicine, Orthopaedics, and Social Medicine, Department of Epidemiology, Gillings School of Global Public Health, The University of North Carolina at Chapel Hill, Chapel Hill, North Carolina

BRIGITTA J. CINTRON, DMSc, PA-C
Doctor of Medical Science, Master of Physician Assistant Studies, Assistant Professor, Florida State University, College of Medicine, School of Physician Assistant Practice, Tallahassee, Florida

TERESA M. CROUT, MD, FACR
Division of Rheumatology, University of Mississippi Medical Center, Jackson, Mississippi

KRISTIN M. D'SILVA, MD
Graduate Assistant, Division of Rheumatology, Allergy, and Immunology, Massachusetts General Hospital, Boston, Massachusetts

ATUL DEODHAR, MD, FRCP
Professor of Medicine, Oregon Health & Science University, Portland, Oregon

JOAN DOBACK, MHP, PA-C
Chief PA, Department of Orthopedics, Bone Health Coordinator, Waterbury Health, Waterbury, Connecticut, USA; Adjunct Clinical Professor, Department of Physician Assistant Studies, Quinnipiac University, North Haven, Connecticut; Adjunct Clinical Professor, Department of Public Health and Community Medicine, Tufts University, Boston, Massachusetts

ARIADNE V. EBEL, DO
Rheumatology Fellow, Division of Rheumatology and Immunology, University of Nebraska Medical Center, Omaha, Nebraska; UCHealth Greeley Hospital, Greeley, Colorado

MICHAEL G. FEELY, MD
Assistant Professor, Department of Internal Medicine, Division of Rheumatology, University of Nebraska Medical Center, Omaha, Nebraska

KATIE F. HUFFMAN, MA
Osteoarthritis Action Alliance, Thurston Arthritis Research Center, The University of North Carolina at Chapel Hill, Chapel Hill, North Carolina

ANAND KUMTHEKAR, MBBS
Assistant Professor of Medicine, Montefiore Medical Center, Albert Einstein College of Medicine, Bronx, New York

DAY S. LENNEP, MD, FACP, FACR
Division of Rheumatology, University of Mississippi Medical Center, Jackson, Mississippi

VIKAS MAJITHIA, MD, MPH, FACP, FACR
Division of Rheumatology, University of Mississippi Medical Center, Jackson, Mississippi

JOAN McTIGUE, PA-C, MS
VA Medical Center and University of Florida, Division of Rheumatology, Gainesville, Florida

AMANDA E. NELSON, MD, MSCR
Associate Professor of Medicine, Osteoarthritis Action Alliance, Thurston Arthritis Research Center, Department of Medicine, The University of North Carolina at Chapel Hill, Chapel Hill, North Carolina

JAMES R. O'DELL, MD, MACP, MACR
Stokes-Shackleford Professor and Vice-Chair of Internal Medicine, Chief, Division of Rheumatology and Immunology, University of Nebraska Medical Center, Omaha Veterans Affairs, Omaha, Nebraska

RICHARD POPE, MPAS, PA-C, DFAAPA, CPAAPA
Retired Rheumatology PA, Department of Rheumatology, Nuvance Health, Danbury, Connecticut; Adjunct Clinical Professor, Department of Physician Assistant Studies, Quinnipiac University, North Haven, Connecticut; Adjunct Clinical Professor, University of Bridgeport, Bridgeport, Connecticut; Invited Guest Lecturer, Yale University School of Medicine, New Haven, Connecticut

CARRIE SCHREIBMAN, MSN, FNP
Instructor, Division of Arthritis and Rheumatic Diseases, Oregon Health & Science University, Portland, Oregon

BARBARA A. SLUSHER, MSW, PA-C
Supervisor, Advanced Practice Providers, MD Anderson Cancer Center, Galveston and League City, League City, Texas

BENJAMIN J SMITH, DMSc, PA-C, DFAAPA
Director of Didactic Education, Assistant Professor, Florida State University College of Medicine, School of Physician Assistant Practice, Tallahassee, Florida; Rheumatology Physician Assistant, McIntosh Clinic, PC, Thomasville, Georgia

TINA H. THORNHILL, PharmD, FASCP, BCGP
Campbell University College of Pharmacy & Health Sciences, Buies Creek, North Carolina

TRACEY B. WRIGHT, MD
Associate Professor of Pediatrics, Division of Rheumatology, Department of Pediatrics, UT Southwestern Medical Center, Dallas, Texas

Contents

The immune system is complex conglomeration of cells, organs, chemicals, and processes designed to protect the self from foreign substances. The immune system is organized into 2 synergistic main branches, innate and adaptive immunity. Autoimmunity is an immune response against self-antigens normally present within the body of the host and the pathogenetic basis of most rheumatic diseases. Autoimmunity is associated with imbalance between pathogenic and the regulatory factors and depends on the inheritance of susceptibility genes and subsequent triggering events. The exact roles of these factors remain unclear in individual diseases/syndromes and subject of further understanding.

There is one thing in medicine that has not changed over the millennia and that is the human body. Likewise, the most important instrument in medicine that a clinician uses on a daily basis is critical thinking, supported by our powerful sense of observation. It is important to understand this concept because it is central to the task of performing a comprehensive history and physical examination and, ultimately, culminating in an accurate diagnosis. This is true for any medical specialty, but particularly important for the specialty of rheumatology because rheumatic diseases are complex and can involve multiple organ systems.

Affecting over 32 million US adults, osteoarthritis (OA) is a complex and serious disease that warrants particular clinical attention given its extensive patient and economic burden, combined with its connection to other chronic conditions and the fact that there is currently no cure. The most effective management and prevention strategies for OA require a partnership between providers and patients, pairing clinical care with patient self-management activities such as physical activity, weight loss, education, and injury prevention.

weakness and poor muscular endurance. Extramuscular manifestations are common and may affect the skin, lungs, gastrointestinal tract, and heart. Myositis-specific antibodies aid in the classification of patients and correlate with specific clinical phenotypes. Corticosteroids and immunosuppressive medications are the mainstay of treatment, although exercise recently has been shown to be an integral part of the management of IIMs.

Osteoporosis is the most common bone disease and has become a major public health problem. It is characterized by low bone mass, deterioration of bone tissue, disruption of bone architecture, compromised bone strength, and an increase in fracture risk. It is a silent disease until it leads to fracture. Osteoporosis exacts both an enormous financial and human toll. It is estimated that 10.2 million people in the United States have osteoporosis, and another 43 million have osteopenia or low bone mass. The cost of treating osteoporotic fractures in the United States is estimated to increase to $25.3 billion by 2025.

The term axial spondylarthritis (AxSpA) includes ankylosing spondylitis and nonradiographic axSpA. The hallmark feature of ankylosing spondylitis is definitive evidence of radiographic sacroiliitis, whereas nonradiographic axSpA has no definitive radiographic sacroiliitis but there is sacroiliitis on MRI. Inflammatory back pain is a classical feature of axSpA along with certain extra-axial features. Early identification and referral improves outcomes in axSpA. Physician assistants and primary care providers play a pivotal role in early recognition or suspicion of axSpA, and ensuring appropriate referrals. This narrative provides a general review of axSpA, clinical clues to diagnose axSpA, imaging modalities used, and available treatment options.

Psoriatic arthritis (PsA) presents a myriad of challenges for each patient to manage. With disease penetration extending to various joint and organ locations, every patient with PsA may present a bit differently. Keeping in mind the effect of disease and its management on the patient's daily life is essential. Associated comorbidities exist with PsA that can have a significant effect on the patient's prognosis and quality of life. This article examines the specifics of PsA, its evaluation, diagnosis, and management while keeping the patient's perspective at the forefront of the discussion.

Systemic sclerosis is a progressive multisystem disease characterized by autoimmunity, endothelial cell dysfunction, and excessive fibrosis in the skin and internal organs. Systemic sclerosis is divided into limited and diffuse cutaneous disease based on the presence of skin fibrosis distal to the elbows and knees (limited) or proximal to the elbows and knees (diffuse). Pharmacologic treatment is directed at the underlying manifestations of the disease (eg, mycophenolate mofetil for diffuse skin thickening and symptomatic progressive interstitial lung disease, proton pump inhibitors for gastroesophageal reflux disease, and calcium channel blockers for Raynaud phenomenon).

Heather Benham and Tracey B. Wright

This article highlights the generalized impact of pediatric rheumatic disease including disturbed growth and development, negative psychosocial implications, altered family dynamics, and risk of morbidities in adulthood. Current research efforts are also discussed. A review of juvenile idiopathic arthritis (JIA) includes diagnostic and classification criteria, incidence and prevalence data, common symptoms, disease-specific evaluation, disease activity measurements, brief review of treatment, and common JIA mimickers. A review of scleroderma includes similar components with a focus on localized scleroderma, the form more common in children.

Heather Benham and Tracey B. Wright

Overview of Pediatric Rheumatology: Part Two highlights systemic lupus erythematosus in childhood, including epidemiology, clinical features, measures of disease activity, damage, and quality as well as approaches to medical management. In addition, a review of juvenile dermatomyositis includes epidemiology, diagnostic criteria, clinical manifestations and assessments, prognostic indicators, and medical management as well as disease course and outcomes. Brief reviews of vasculitidies and autoinflammatory syndromes in childhood are also included.

PHYSICIAN ASSISTANT CLINICS

SERIES OF RELATED INTEREST

Primary Care: Clinics in Office Practice
https://www.primarycare.theclinics.com/

THE CLINICS ARE AVAILABLE ONLINE!
Access your subscription at:
www.theclinics.com

Foreword
PA Week

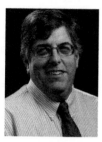

James A. Van Rhee, MS, PA-C
Consulting Editor

As I write this foreword, we are celebrating PA week. National PA Day was first cele-brated on October 6, 1987; yes, it was only a single day at first. This date is the date of the first graduation in 1967 and is also the birthday of Dr Eugene Stead Jr.

As we honor all the physician assistants (PAs) providing care, educating future PAs, and providing support to PAs and patients in a wide variety of settings, please take a moment or two and thank the PA faculty who helped you on this journey, thank the PA mentors who have aided in your growth as a PA, and thank all the other members of the health care team that you work with to provide care to patients.

The PA profession has always been about collaborative practice and team-oriented care. During this COVID-19 pandemic, these concepts have proven to be even more important. So, thank you to all the PAs, all 139,000 plus, providing care every day and improving the lives of those they care for.

This issue of *Physician Assistant Clinics*, with guest editor, Benjamin Smith, provides an excellent review of the rheumatologic disorders. This issue takes the reader from the immunologic basics of disease by Majithia, to the evaluation of the rheumatology patient by Slusher. All the common disorders are covered from osteoarthritis by Huffman, rheumatoid arthritis by O'Dell and Ebel, systemic lupus by Smith, and crystal arthritides by McTigue. But we don't just cover the more common disorders in this issue. Schreibman provides an excellent review of fibromyalgia; Feely explains the in-flammatory myopathies, and Kumthekar and Deodhar review the spondyloarthritis. Cintron covers psoriatic arthritis, and Bolster and D'Silva discuss systemic sclerosis. Pope and Doback cover the latest information related to the diagnosis and treatment of osteoporosis, and Benham and Wright review pediatric rheumatology.

Physician Assist Clin 6 (2021) xv–xvi
https://doi.org/10.1016/j.cpha.2020.10.002
2405-7991/21/© 2020 Published by Elsevier Inc.

physicianassistant.theclinics.com

I hope you enjoy this issue. Our next issue will cover topics in surgery.

James A. Van Rhee, MS, PA-C
Yale School of Medicine
Yale Physician Assistant Online Program
100 Church Street South, Suite A230
New Haven, CT 06519, USA

E-mail address:
james.vanrhee@yale.edu

Website:
http://www.paonline.yale.edu

Preface

Rheumatology: Opportunities Await to Do Much Good!

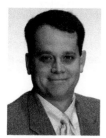

Benjamin J Smith, DMSc, PA-C, DFAAPA
Editor

When I began working in rheumatology as a physician assistant (PA) over 20 years ago, I could not have imagined the opportunities that lie in store. In part, these opportunities have come because of many years of scientific discovery (begun long before I was born) that is resulting in medical advances now. Our understanding and approach to rheumatic disease have further evolved during my short career. We seek to recognize and treat rheumatic disease earlier in its course. We monitor those with rheumatic disease diligently. We have an armamentarium of nonpharmacologic and pharmacologic modalities that can be chosen in accordance with each patient's unique experience.

These opportunities have provided (and continue to lead to) much professional and personal development. Most of these opportunities have come through interactions with persons with rheumatic disease. It is truly a humbling privilege to meet someone at a time when they are experiencing symptoms that often occur for unknown reasons. Although as clinicians we do not have all the answers, we can share medical knowledge and guidance at a time that a person cannot totally help themselves. Working together to make treatment decisions is an awesome task. Much joy and happiness are felt when you see someone rise from a wheelchair or a hospital bed. I am grateful to be a member of the rheumatology community.

For some, rheumatology is seen as mysterious and hard-to-diagnose conditions, laboratory that seems to use every letter of the alphabet in their name, and medications that are not commonly prescribed. Our hope, as you take the opportunity to consider and digest the contents of this issue of *Physician Assistant Clinics*, is that you will gain much by way of review and recognition of new medical knowledge in your pursuit of providing high-quality and compassionate patient care. Remember, as my rheumatology mentor and friend Dr Victor M. McMillan often reminds me, the art of medicine is vital in our work as clinicians. In other words, it is putting the pieces of the rheumatic disease puzzle together to see the picture that is in front of us.

Physician Assist Clin 6 (2021) xvii–xviii
https://doi.org/10.1016/j.cpha.2020.10.001
2405-7991/21/© 2020 Published by Elsevier Inc.

I wish to express my sincerest gratitude, appreciation, and admiration to the authors of the insightful articles contained in this issue focused on rheumatology. One opportunity of which I have been afforded is to meet and build friendships with rheumatology experts around the world. The authors of the articles in this issue are a representation of the many dedicated professionals in the specialty of rheumatology. I consider the authors of these articles to be my esteemed colleagues and friends. You will recognize the authors to be of varied disciplines and backgrounds. The care of persons with rheumatic disease is most optimally accomplished through interdisciplinary teams as represented by the authors of this issue. PAs are vital members of the rheumatology team!

Enjoy those things that you will discover in the pages of this issue. My hope is that you will recognize the opportunities that you have to increase and apply your medical knowledge to better serve those for whom you provide care.

Much success to each of you,

Benjamin J Smith, DMSc, PA-C, DFAAPA
Florida State University College of Medicine
School of Physician Assistant Practice
1115 West Call Street
Tallahassee, FL 32306-4300, USA

E-mail address:
benjamin.smith@med.fsu.edu

Immunology Basics of Rheumatic Disease

Teresa M. Crout, MD*, Day S. Lennep, MD, Vikas Majithia, MD, MPH

KEYWORDS

- Immunology • Rheumatology • Autoimmunity • Major histocompatibility complex
- Rheumatic illnesses • Innate immunity • Adaptive immunity • Tolerance

KEY POINTS

- Autoimmunity is immune responsiveness against self-antigens and plays a central role in causation of rheumatic illnesses.
- Autoimmune diseases are pathologic conditions associated with an abnormal adaptive immunity response directed against an antigen within the body of the host.
- Principal factors in the development of autoimmunity are the inheritance of susceptibility genes and a trigger usually environmental in predisposed individuals.
- The development of autoimmune disease depends on an imbalance between pathogenic factors generated by autoreactive T cells and B cells and the regulatory factors that normally control the immune response.
- Manifestations of autoimmune rheumatic diseases usually involve the development of inflammation and its consequences and may also be associated with autoantibodies.

INTRODUCTION AND BACKGROUND

The immune system refers to a collection of cells, chemicals, and processes that function to protect the skin, respiratory passages, intestinal tract, and other areas from foreign antigens, such as microbes (organisms such as bacteria, fungi, and parasites), viruses, cancer cells, and toxins. The primary function of the immune system is to protect the body from a foreign insult, primarily infection. To be able to perform the function, the immune system has evolved into its current complex form with a variety of components, compartments, and processes.

Beyond the structural and chemical barriers that protect us from infection, the immune system can be simplistically viewed as having 2 lines of defense: innate immunity and adaptive immunity. Innate and adaptive immunity are not mutually exclusive mechanisms of host defense, but rather are complementary, with defects in either system resulting in host vulnerability such as immunodeficiency or inappropriate

Division of Rheumatology, University of Mississippi Medical Center, 2500 North State Street, Jackson, MS 39216, USA
* Corresponding author. L-002, 2500 North State Street, Jackson, MS 39216.
E-mail address: tcrout@umc.edu

Physician Assist Clin 6 (2021) 1–14
https://doi.org/10.1016/j.cpha.2020.08.002
2405-7991/21/© 2020 Elsevier Inc. All rights reserved.

physicianassistant.theclinics.com

responses such as autoimmunity. Autoimmunity involves the loss of normal immune homeostasis such that the organism produces an abnormal response to its own tissue. The hallmark of autoimmunity is the presence of self-reactive T cells, autoantibodies, and inflammation. Most inflammatory rheumatologic diseases result from autoimmunity.

This article aims to provide a basic introduction to the main components and function of the immune system and its role in both health and disease with an emphasis on its role in rheumatic disease.

CELLS AND TISSUES OF THE IMMUNE SYSTEM

Numerous cells exist as a part of the immune system and are located in several different tissues. They each serve different roles to help with host defense. First, there are lymphocytes, separated into T lymphocytes and B lymphocytes, which can be found in lymphoid organs and nonlymphoid tissues. Their goal is to identify foreign antigens and alert the body to use its adaptive immune responses.[1] More detail about lymphocytes is provided elsewhere in this article.

There are phagocytes, which function to consume microbes and kill them. Two main kinds exist: neutrophils and macrophages. Neutrophils are short lived, the most abundant, and are also known as polymorphonuclear leukocytes. Polymorphonuclear leukocytes are typically found in response to bacterial and fungal infections and are usually the first to respond to infection. In contrast, macrophages have multiple functions. They begin as monocytes, which will then later differentiate into macrophages once they enter into extravascular tissue. As a macrophage, they will phagocytose microbes, similar to neutrophils, but they live longer and are less abundant. They will also eliminate dead tissues and start the process of repairing tissue. Macrophages play a role in displaying antigens to lymphocytes, specifically T lymphocytes, and thus also fall under the category of antigen-presenting cells (APCs). Monocytes can also differentiate into dendritic cells. Dendritic cells' main function is to serve as APCs; they exist to recognize and catch microbes, and in turn present them to lymphocytes.[1]

Mast cells, which can be found in the connective tissue surrounding blood vessels, serve to alert and recruit other leukocytes by releasing various cytokines.[2] They also secrete enzymes that can neutralize microbial toxins.[1] Basophils act in a similar manner, although they are found in the circulation. Both mast cells and basophils are 2 important cells in starting the inflammatory cascade and play a large role in symptoms of allergic disease.[1,2] Another cell involved with allergy mechanism are eosinophils. These cells are called granulocytes and are important in the destroying parasites that can be too large to phagocytose.

Natural killer (NK) cells play a large role in cleaning up by killing infected cells. They do this by eventually inducing apoptosis of infected cells. NK cells also produce cytokines to recruit APCs and help to make them more effective at killing microbes. Last, innate lymphoid cells are similar to lymphocytes in their function, but they do not contain something call T-cell antigen receptors. There are 3 major groups, which are defined by the type of cytokine they secrete and help guide immune responses.[2] **Table 1** summarizes the main types of immune cells and their functions.

The tissues of the immune system can be broken down into 2 types: generative (or primary) lymphoid organs and peripheral (or secondary) lymphoid organs.

The generative lymphoid organs include the bone marrow and the thymus. These organs are where the T and B lymphocytes are generated, mature, and gain the function to respond to antigens. The peripheral lymphoid organs include the lymph

Table 1
Characteristics of leukocytes involved in innate immunity[1]

Cell	Image	Location	Function(s)	Lifespan
Neutrophil		Circulate in blood, migrate to tissue	Phagocytosis Degranulation	Several hours to a few days
Macrophage		Circulate in blood, migrate to tissue	Phagocytosis Antigen presentation	Months to years
Dendritic cell		Epithelial tissue, migrates to lymph nodes	Antigen presentation	Few days
Mast cells		Connective tissues, mucous membranes	Cytokine release Neutralize microbial toxins Degranulation	Months to years

(continued on next page)

Table 1 (continued)

Cell	Image	Location	Function(s)	Lifespan
Basophils		Circulate in blood, migrate to tissue	Cytokine release Degranulation	Few hours to few days
Eosinophils		Circulate in blood, migrate to tissue	Cytokine release Degranulation	Eight to 12 days
NK cells		Circulate in blood, migrate to tissue	Destruction of infected cells Cytokine release	Seven to 10 days

Adapted from Warrington, R., Watson, W., Kim, H.L. et al. An introduction to immunology and immunopathology. All Asth Clin Immun 7, S1 (2011). https://doi.org/10.1186/1710-1492-7-S1-S1; with permission.

nodes, spleen, and mucosal and cutaneous immune tissues. They serve as a location for lymphocytes to interact with antigens and help to develop adaptive immune responses.[1]

INNATE AND ADAPTIVE IMMUNITY

The immune system is organized into 2 main branches, innate immunity and adaptive immunity. The purpose is to recognize and destroy foreign invaders. Innate immunity works quickly and is not specific to a certain pathogen. Adaptive immunity takes longer, is more targeted, and can have lasting memory for long-term immunity (**Fig. 1, Table 2**).

Innate immunity is the body's first line of defense against pathogens. Sometimes innate immunity is also called natural immunity, and it is genetically determined at birth. It works immediately and within 24 hours. It is made up of a variety of different components including complement, C-reactive protein, mannan-binding lectin, NK cells, mast cells, macrophages, neutrophils, dendritic cells, eosinophils, basophils, mast cells, natural antibodies, epithelia, and fibroblasts. Skin and the mucous membranes work as physical barriers to block invaders in the innate immune system. Pathogen recognition is broad, to catch all types of invaders, working by recognizing structures common to types of microbes. It does not remember the pathogen when it is through (it does not have memory) and does not become permanently changed once it has been exposed to an antigen.[1]

Innate immunity destroys or removes pathogens by a variety of mechanisms. This process may involve direct cell lysis, such as with viruses, opsonization by antibodies or complement and microbial killing by phagocytic cells. The innate immune system also functions to present antigens, secrete chemokines to recruit more innate and adaptive immunity cells, and activate T and B cells.

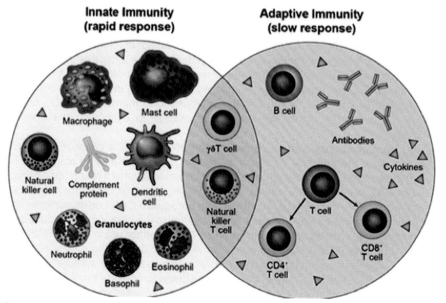

Fig. 1. Innate versus adaptive immune responses. (*From* Dranoff, G. Cytokines in cancer pathogenesis and cancer therapy. Nat Rev Cancer. 4, 11–22 (2004); with permission.)

Table 2
Comparison of innate and adaptive immunity

	Innate Immunity	Adaptive Immunity
Response	Fast, <24 h	Slower, >24 h
Germline	Coded	Rearranged
Specific to each individual organism?	No	Yes
Memory?	No	Yes
Examples of components	Complement, C-reactive protein, mannan-binding lectin, NK cells, mast cells, macrophages, neutrophils, dendritic cells, eosinophils, basophils, mast cells, epithelia, fibroblasts	T cells B cells Lymphokines

From Noss, EH. Basic Science for the Rheumatologist: The Brigham Board Review in Rheumatology, Brigham and Women's Hospital. Oakstone Publishing, LLC. May 1, 2014.

The innate immune system recognizes pathogens because of structures specific to microbes, which are generally called pathogen-associated molecular patterns (PAMPs). The PAMP structures on the microbes are recognized by the receptors from the cells of the innate immune system, called pattern recognition receptors. Examples of PAMPs include lipopolysaccharides (from gram-negative bacteria), peptidoglycan (from gram-positive bacteria), and DNA and RNA (from viruses). Examples of pattern recognition receptors include toll-like receptors, nucleotide oligomerization domain-like receptors, collectins, lectins, and pentraxins. In a patient with gout, urate crystals act like PAMPs, which will activate nucleotide oligomerization domain-like receptors to try to get rid of the unwanted substance.[3,4]

Adaptive immunity, in contrast, will start to work slower than innate immunity and is also sometimes referred to as specific or acquired immunity. If the innate immunity system cannot completely take care of the pathogen, the adaptive immunity will respond. Its response may take 24 hours or more, but it can distinguish 1 organism from another. B cells, T cells, and lymphokines (interleukins) make up the composition of adaptive immunity, which has the ability to form memory cells. On repeat exposure, the memory cells will work more quickly to extinguish the specific pathogen.[1,3]

If the innate immunity system cannot handle the invader, a cascade of events takes place for the adaptive immunity system to be stimulated and respond. The pathogen becomes endocytosed because it is bound to a pattern recognition receptor on an APC. Take a dendritic cell (a type of APC) for example; it becomes activated when the antigen is internalized, and it will then upregulate CCR7 on its surface. This process will cause it to leave its area and move toward a chemokine produced by lymphoid tissue, where it will be presented to T cells (either using major histocompatibility complex [MHC] class I or class II molecules, depending on the antigen). The APC also will upregulate costimulatory molecules on its surface, such as CD80/CD86. A perfect cascade of events takes place to activate the T cell and ultimately result in stimulation of the adaptive immunity process; an APC presents the MHC class molecule with the antigen to the T-cell receptor while the costimulatory molecules bind.[3]

ANTIGEN PRESENTATION, T-CELL–MEDIATED IMMUNITY, AND B-CELL–MEDIATED IMMUNITY

Antigen presentation starts with an APC; examples include histiocytes (connective tissue), monocytes (blood), alveolar macrophages (lung), Kupffer cells (liver), microglia (central nervous system), dendritic cells (lymphoid, mucous membranes, solid organs), Langerhans cells (skin, or dendritic cells), and B lymphocytes (lymph nodes). Each APC has a MHC that encodes a HLA. MHCs are either class I, II, or III and their role is to help present a peptide antigen to a T cell. See **Table 3**, which compares MHC HLA class I and class II molecules; they are on different types of cells, will help to present different size antigens, vary in which type of antigen, and are recognized by different types of T cells.[3]

There is a large pool of T and B cells in the body, each with unique receptor specificity. In T cells, the T-cell receptor has either a CD4 or CD8 molecule, which determines its ultimate function. The B cell's receptor is the immunoglobulin it has made on its surface.

A 2-step signaling event is required to stimulate B and T cells. For T cells, they are first stimulated when a microbial product is phagocytosed by an APC, processed into a peptide, and loaded onto an MHC molecule to be presented to the T cell.

For B cells, they are first activated when their surface immunoglobulin becomes cross-linked by an antigen. The second signal after each initial activation is induced by signs of inflammation, which activates the innate immunity system and pattern recognition receptors leading to upregulation of cell surface costimulatory molecules and cytokine activation. Importantly, signal one without signal 2 will lead to anergy or lack of response. For example, in relation to activation of a T-cell response, an APC presents an antigen on its MHC molecule and it is recognized by the T-cell receptor as signal 1. Signal 2 occurs at the same time when the microbial products are activating pattern recognition receptors and stimulating upregulation of B7 on the APC, which binds to CD28 on the T cell.

Clonal expansion happens when this process occurs, and the T or B cell can then proliferate. Often, they can then mature into effector cells. Effector T cells can cause direct cell lysis (viruses), stimulate B-cell responses and activate the innate immune system. As an example of effector T-cell response, CD4$^+$ T cells can differentiate into different classes of T helper (Th) cells, Th1, Th2, Th17, and T regulatory cells. Each of these T helper cells will secrete different cytokines and ultimately have variable functions in the immune response. Th1 secretes interferon gamma, helping with defense against viruses and intracellular bacteria. Th2 cells secrete IL-4, IL-5,

Table 3		
Comparison of MHC HLA class I and II		
	MHC HLA Class I	**MHC HLA Class II**
Type of cell	On all nucleated cells, platelets	On B cells, macrophages, dendritic cells, some activated T cells, some cells after being induced such as synovial cells
Antigen (peptide fragment)	Intracellular, for example, viruses, tumor antigens	Extracellular, then phagocytosed or endocytosed into lysosomal compartments, for example, bacteria
T-cell recognition	CD8$^+$ T cell	CD4$^+$ T cell
Response	Cell-mediated killing	T-cell–induced phagocytosis and/or antibody response

and IL-13, killing parasites. Th17 secretes IL-17, IL-21, and IL-22, working against extracellular bacteria and fungi.[3] T regulatory cells play a role in immune tolerance, as will be discussed elsewhere in this article. Effector B cells become plasma cells, which secrete antibodies. Some B and T cells will become memory cells, providing immunity to past infections[3] (**Fig. 2**).

Cytokines

Cytokines are small proteins, peptides, and glycoproteins that act intermediary in cell-to-cell signaling and communications.[5] Cytokines are produced by a broad range of cells, including immune cells like macrophages, B lymphocytes, T lymphocytes, and mast cells, as well as endothelial cells, fibroblasts, and various stromal cells; a given cytokine may be produced by more than 1 type of cell. Cytokines enable immune cells

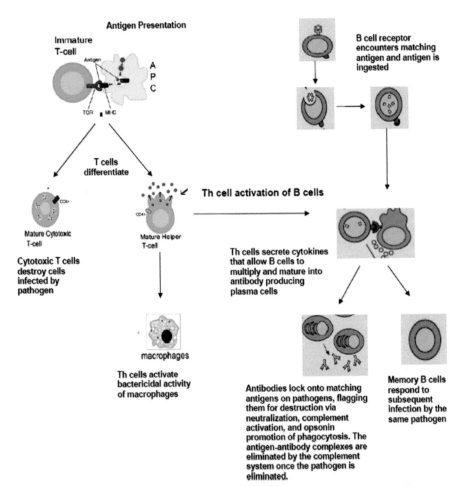

Fig. 2. Adaptive immunity: T-cell and B-cell activation and function. MHC, major histocompatibility complex; TCR, T-cell receptor. (*From* Warrington R, Watson W, Kim HL, Antonetti FR. An introduction to immunology and immunopathology. Allergy Asthma Clin Immunol. 2011;7 Suppl 1(Suppl 1):S1. Published 2011 Nov 10. https://doi.org/10.1186/1710-1492-7-S1-S1; with permission.)

to communicate with one another by either direct contact or through the secretion of soluble mediators. They play an integral role in the initiation, perpetuation, and subsequent downregulation of the immune response.[5] Cytokines include chemokines, interferons, interleukins, lymphokines, tumor necrosis factors, and some other proteins.[5,6]

ROLE OF CYTOKINES IN INFLAMMATION

Poorly regulated inflammatory responses and tissue damage as a result of inflammation are often immunopathologic features of autoimmune diseases.[6] Inflammation is usually an integral part of the normal host response to infection, injury, or stress and necessary to fight back and remove a pathogen or lead to healing. Uncontrolled and unchecked inflammation leads to a chronic inflammatory response and development and perpetuation of autoimmune diseases.[6] Owing to an aberrant immune response, there is recruitment of inflammatory cells and overproduction of inflammatory cytokines (such as IL-1, IL-6, and tumor necrosis factor-alpha), which leads to the initiation and perpetuation of the tissue and organ damage and various manifestations of the autoimmune diseases.[6]

NORMAL AND ABERRANT IMMUNE RESPONSES: TOLERANCE AND AUTOIMMUNITY

One of the remarkable properties of the normal immune system is that it can react to an enormous variety of microbes but does not react against the individual's own (self) antigens, that is, antigens normally present within the body of the host.[1] The lack of responsiveness to self-antigens is called immunologic tolerance.[1] The immune cells are constantly exposed to the self and pathogenic non-self antigens primarily microbes and a normal immune system is able to differentiate these 2 and react appropriately. When the normal mechanisms of tolerance break down, it leads to autoimmunity and autoimmune diseases.[1]

MECHANISMS FOR IMMUNOLOGIC TOLERANCE

- Central T- and B-Cell Tolerance: Deletion of self-reactive T cells in the thymus during the development process.[1,7]
- Peripheral T- and B-Cell Tolerance:
  - Anergy: Works by inducing unresponsive state of T cells that have encountered their specific antigen without costimulatory signals.[8]
  - Immunologic Ignorance: Lack of a productive encounter between the T cell and its corresponding peptide/MHC complex on an APC.[9]
  - Regulation by Inhibitory Receptors: There are inhibitory receptors and pathways on autoreactive immune cells, which can prevent development and propagation of self-reactive T cells.[1,10]
  - Suppression by Regulatory Cells: There are regulatory T cells, B cells, and NK cells that inhibit responses to self-antigens.[10]
  - Apoptosis: Programmed cell death leads to inhibition and clearance of autoreactive cells.[1,10]

AUTOIMMUNITY

Autoimmunity is defined as an immune response against self-antigens. It involves the loss of normal immune tolerance, leading to the abnormal immune response to its own cells and tissues. The hallmark of autoimmunity is the presence of self-reactive T cells, autoantibodies, and inflammation.

CLINICAL CORRELATION WITH RHEUMATIC DISEASES

As mentioned elsewhere in this article, defects or malfunctions in either the innate or adaptive immune response can provoke illness or disease. Such disorders are generally caused by an overactive immune response (known as hypersensitivity reactions), an inappropriate reaction to self (known as autoimmunity), or ineffective immune responses (known as immunodeficiency).[2] Most of the rheumatic diseases fall into the category of autoimmunity, although the diseases cause its manifestations usually by activating 1 or more of the hypersensitivity reaction pathways.[1,2]

AUTOIMMUNITY AND RHEUMATIC DISEASES

Autoimmune disease is defined as an adaptive immune response against self (autologous) antigens; that is, antigens normally present within the body of the host.[2,6] It is an important cause of inflammatory rheumatologic diseases, with a prevalence of 2% to 5% of the population in developed countries.

Different autoimmune diseases may be organ specific, affecting only 1 or a few organs, or systemic, with widespread tissue injury and clinical manifestations. A number of pathways of cellular, tissue, and organ injury in autoimmune diseases follow 1 or more of hypersensitivity reactions, which may be caused by antibodies against self-antigens or by T cells reactive with self-antigens. The pathologic basis of autoimmunity is usually a specific adaptive autoimmune response that usually continues after the altered self-antigen is eliminated.

Autoimmune disease usually involves both T-cell and B-cell responses directed to a self-antigen. Autoimmunity can also contribute to an ongoing disease by worsening the ongoing process and the pathology.[11]

DEVELOPMENT OF AUTOIMMUNE DISEASES

The principal factors in the development of autoimmunity are the inheritance of susceptibility genes and environmental triggers, such as infections in these predisposed individuals.[1,6,12] It is, however, very clear that we do not know exactly how these genes play a role for sure or what is the actual environmental trigger, if any, in the development of autoimmune rheumatic diseases.

Genetic Basis

Autoimmune diseases have a strong genetic basis and tend to cluster in family members and people with certain susceptibility genes. It is postulated that susceptibility genes interfere with pathways of self-tolerance and lead to the persistence of self-reactive T and B lymphocytes. Stimuli—both environmental and internal—may cause triggering of the autoimmunity by cell and tissue injury leading to inflammation and activation of these self-reactive lymphocytes, resulting in the generation of effector T cells and autoantibodies that are responsible for the autoimmune disease.[1,6]

Environmental Triggers and Role of Infection

The infections are notoriously common triggers for autoimmune disease, but other environmental insults such as injury, sunlight, chemicals, or internal aberrations as in cancer, stress, and surgery also play a role. Infections can provide the requisite antigen by mimicking or altering of self-antigens or by antigen spillage.[13] The infections can also provide an inflammatory milieu via innate immunity that leads to initiation or propagation of autoimmunity. The micro-organisms that generally inhabit body surfaces, including the skin and mucus membranes, also influence both the initiation and progression of an autoimmune response. In individuals, populations of commensal micro-organisms ("microbiota") can profoundly affect the induction of such diseases as inflammatory bowel diseases.[14] An example of infectious agent playing a role in autoimmune disease is Epstein–Barr virus as a potential instigating agent in multiple sclerosis, and systemic lupus erythematosus.[15]

Pathogenetic Mechanisms of Autoimmune Diseases

Despite their diverse etiology, certain pathogenetic mechanisms are common to all autoimmune diseases with most, if not all, involving the adaptive immune response. These diseases require the presence of self-reactive CD4-positive T lymphocytes, barring a few exceptions.

Thymic selection is critical for normal T-cell development and depends on interaction with thymic stromal cells. If the appropriate self-antigens are not properly presented in the thymus, it can result in the development of autoimmune diseases. An example of an abnormality in this process is an altered or mutation in AIRE gene, which can lead to several combinations of autoimmune endocrine diseases, such as autoimmune polyendocrinopathy and candidiasis ectodermal dystrophy.[16]

Another major mechanism is a lack of deletion of self-reactive T cells in the thymus during the development process. There is strong experimental evidence that the deletion of self-reactive lymphocytes occurs in the thymus, and this mechanism seems to be totally effective only for the most prominent systemically expressed antigens, such as those of the major blood groups and histocompatibility complex.[7] By comparison, in the case of most other self-antigens, deletion of self-reactive T cells in the thymus is either lacking or incomplete.[7]

Fortunately, there are mechanisms in the periphery that retard the activation of those self-reactive T cells that escape deletion in the thymus. However, upon exposure to the correct antigen in the right circumstance, the autoimmunity can initiate and progress.

Breakdown in the various mechanisms of peripheral tolerance is well documented in development of autoimmunity:

- Clonal anergy can be terminated by an encounter with appropriate, nonspecific, costimulatory signals from injured tissue and there by initiate autoimmune disease.[8]
- Ignorance can be overcome by changes in antigen availability, such as presentation by an infecting micro-organism.[9] These events can cause autoimmunity and can possibly give rise to autoimmune disease.
- A breakdown in the function of the regulatory T cells, B cells, and NK cells can lead to the development of autoimmune diseases.[10] A heritable defect in the suppressive effects of CD4$^+$ CD25$^+$ Fox P3 regulatory T cells seems to be the mechanism underlying the rare lethal autoimmune human disease.[17]

Whether autoimmune disease will follow an autoimmune response depends on both the quality of the immune response and the availability of the corresponding antigen.

Pathways and Mechanisms Involved in Autoimmune Diseases

Autoantibodies are a common mechanism involved in the initiation and propagation of inflammatory process of autoimmune diseases. Antigens on the surface of circulating cells such as red blood cells, white blood cells, and platelets are exposed to circulating antibodies and damaged or eliminated by autoantibodies by activation of complement, killer T cells, or phagocytes. The autoantibodies against receptors on cell surfaces may lead to activation of the receptor as in Graves' disease or in blocking the neuromuscular transmission in myasthenia gravis or cause damage by activation of complement and phagocytes in antiglomerular basement membrane disease. Enzymes may also be a target of autoantibodies for example, in autoimmune hepatitis and primary biliary cholangitis.[18]

Many other autoimmune diseases are associated with T-cell–mediated immune responses that lead to damage by cytotoxic effector T cells damaging target cells or by producing harmful cytokines or activating macrophages.[19] Carriage of the 1858T variant of the protein tyrosine phosphatase nonreceptor 22 gene (PTPN22) has been linked to T-cell hyperresponsiveness and associated with several autoimmune conditions, including rheumatoid arthritis, systemic lupus erythematosus, Graves' disease, and type 1 diabetes mellitus.[20]

There is also role of innate mechanisms in autoimmunity.[21] There are a number of families of pattern-recognition receptors such as Toll-like receptors, the nucleotide oligomerization domain-like receptors, and the NACHT leucine-rich-repeat proteins.[22] Variants of NACHT leucine-rich-repeat protein 1 are associated with autoimmune disorders that cluster with vitiligo and include rheumatoid arthritis and psoriasis, among others.[23]

T helper 1/T helper 2 dichotomy

In human disease, it is frequently impossible to clearly separate the injury that is due to antibody-mediated from cell-mediated reactions. In general, however, the cell-mediated responses are associated with the Th1 subset of CD4$^+$ T cells and the antibody-mediated mechanisms in general associate with Th2 responses.[24] Thus, sometimes an autoimmune disorder can benefit by a shift from a Th1 to a Th2 response and may be one of the approaches to therapy.

This original, simplistic view of the Th1/Th2 dichotomy is not easily applied to human disease in which both Th1 and Th2 responses are generally evident. It is now evident that a third T-cell subset producing IL-17 (termed Th17) plays a critical role in several autoimmune conditions.[25]

Autoinflammatory Syndromes

The term autoinflammatory syndrome refers to a group of autosomal-predominant inherited disorders that resemble traditional autoimmune diseases, but are distinguished by the absence of a defined adaptive immune response.[26] The prototypic disorders were in a group of hereditary periodic fever syndromes that shared a common involvement of certain specific cytokines such as IL-1 and tumor necrosis factor. Study of these disorders revealed a prominent role for the innate immune system. Mutant NACHT leucine-rich-repeat protein 3, also known as cryopyrin, is linked to 3 inflammatory disorders associated with autosomal dominant inheritance: the familial cold urticaria syndrome, the Muckle–Wells syndrome, and neonatal-onset multisystem inflammatory disease.[27]

SUMMARY

The immune system refers to a collection of cells, organs, chemicals, and processes that function to protect the self from foreign substances, such as microbes, cancer cells, and toxins. To be able to perform their functions, immune system has evolved into current complex form with a variety of components, compartments and processes. The immune system is organized into 2 main branches, innate immunity and adaptive immunity. There is a great deal of synergy between the adaptive immune system and its innate counterpart, and defects in either system can lead to immunopathologic disorders, including autoimmune diseases and immunodeficiencies.

Autoimmunity is defined as an immune response against self (autologous) antigens; that is, antigens normally present within the body of the host. It is an important cause of inflammatory rheumatologic diseases. The development of autoimmune disease depends on an imbalance between pathogenic factors generated by autoreactive T cells and B cells and the regulatory factors that normally control the immune response. Autoimmune diseases are deeply rooted in an abnormal adaptive autoimmune response, but innate immunity also plays a significant role. The principal factors in the development of autoimmunity and rheumatic diseases are the inheritance of susceptibility genes and environmental triggers, such as infections in these predisposed individuals. However, the exact roles of the genetic and environmental factors remain unclear in individual diseases and syndromes and yet to be completely understood.

CLINICS CARE POINTS

- Innate immunity is the primary player in autoinflammatory diseases.
- Principal factors in developing autoimmunity are not fully understood, but genetic predisposition and environmental triggers are thought to play a role.
- Understanding the immunologic basis of rheumatic diseases has led to major breakthroughs in the management of these diseases by targeting various cells, receptors, cytokines and processes involved.
- Examples include: Targeted therapies block TNF, interleukin-6 and Janus kinases to treat rheumatoid arthritis, Abatacept blocks the 2nd step in 2-step signaling for T-cell activation leading to efficacy in treatment of rheumatoid arthritis and psoriatic arthritis and inhibitors of interleukin-17 are being used to treat spondyloarthropathies and psoriatic arthritis.

DISCLOSURE

The authors have nothing to disclose.

REFERENCES

1. Abbas AK, Lichtman AH, Pillai S. Basic immunology: functions and disorders of the immune system. 5th edition. St. Louis (MO): Elsevier; 2016.
2. Marshall JS, Warrington R, Watson W, et al. An introduction to immunology and immunopathology. Allergy Asthma Clin Immunol 2018;14:49.
3. Dranoff G. Cytokines in cancer pathogenesis and cancer therapy. Nat Rev Cancer 2004;4:11–22.
4. West SG. Rheumatology secrets. 3rd edition. Elsevier; 2015. p. 24–38.
5. An introduction to immunology and immunopathology - Scientific Figure on ResearchGate. Available at: https://www.researchgate.net/figure/Adaptive-immunity-T-cell-and-B-cell-activation-and-function-APC-antigen-presenting_fig2_51875109. Accessed February 28, 2020.
6. Davidson A, Diamond B. Autoimmune diseases. N Engl J Med 2001;345(5):340.
7. Dighiero G, Rose NR. Critical self-epitopes are key to the understanding of self-tolerance and autoimmunity. Immunol Today 1999;20(9):423.
8. Nossal GJ. A purgative mastery. Nature 2001;412(6848):685.
9. Kamradt T, Mitchison NA. Tolerance and autoimmunity. N Engl J Med 2001; 344(9):655.
10. King C, Ilic A, Koelsch K, et al. Homeostatic expansion of T cells during immune insufficiency generates autoimmunity. Cell 2004;117(2):265.

11. Rose NR. Viral myocarditis. Curr Opin Rheumatol 2016;28(4):383.
12. Miller FW, Pollard KM, Parks CG, et al. Criteria for environmentally associated autoimmune diseases. J Autoimmun 2012;39(4):253.
13. Rose NR. Negative selection, epitope mimicry and autoimmunity. Curr Opin Immunol 2017;49:51.
14. Elson CO, Alexander KL. Host-microbiota interactions in the intestine. Dig Dis 2015;33(2):131–6.
15. Ascherio A, Munger KL. EBV and Autoimmunity. Curr Top Microbiol Immunol 2015;390(Pt 1):365.
16. De Martino L, Capalbo D, Improda N, et al. APECED: a paradigm of complex interactions between genetic background and susceptibility factors. Front Immunol 2013;4:331.
17. Wildin RS, Smyk-Pearson S, Filipovich AH. Clinical and molecular features of the immunodysregulation, polyendocrinopathy, enteropathy, X linked (IPEX) syndrome. J Med Genet 2002;39(8):537.
18. Bogdanos DP, Dalekos GN. Enzymes as target antigens of liver-specific autoimmunity: the case of cytochromes P450s. Curr Med Chem 2008;15(22):2285.
19. Ueda H, Howson JM, Esposito L, et al. Association of the T-cell regulatory gene CTLA4 with susceptibility to autoimmune disease. Nature 2003;423(6939):506.
20. Lee YH, Rho YH, Choi SJ, et al. The PTPN22 C1858T functional polymorphism and autoimmune diseases–a meta-analysis. Rheumatology (Oxford) 2007;46(1):49.
21. Gregersen PK. Modern genetics, ancient defenses, and potential therapies. N Engl J Med 2007;356(12):1263.
22. Meylan E, Tschopp J, Karin M. Intracellular pattern recognition receptors in the host response. Nature 2006;442(7098):39.
23. Jin Y, Mailloux CM, Gowan K. NALP1 in vitiligo-associated multiple autoimmune disease. N Engl J Med 2007;356(12):1216.
24. Emmi L, Romagnani S. Role of Th1 and Th2 cells in autoimmunity. In: Rose NR, Mackay IR, editors. The autoimmune diseases. San Diego (CA): Academic Press; 2006. p. 83–101.
25. Martinez GJ, Nurieva RI, Yang XO, et al. Regulation and function of proinflammatory TH17 cells. Ann N Y Acad Sci 2008;1143:188.
26. Park H, Bourla AB, Kastner DL, et al. Lighting the fires within: the cell biology of autoinflammatory diseases. Nat Rev Immunol 2012;12(8):570.
27. Stojanov S, Kastner DL. Familial autoinflammatory diseases: genetics, pathogenesis and treatment. Curr Opin Rheumatol 2005;17(5):586.

Identifying Patterns

Linking History, Review of Systems, and Physical Examination in Rheumatic Musculoskeletal Diseases

Barbara A. Slusher, MSW, PA-C

KEYWORDS

- Rheumatic musculoskeletal disease • History • Review of systems
- Physical examination

KEY POINTS

- The rheumatology health professional's most valuable tool for diagnosing and treating rheumatic musculoskeletal diseases is the comprehensive history and physical examination.
- Review of systems is the thread that links the subjective (patient-centered history) with the objective (provider-focused observation and physical examination).
- These 3 components are the cornerstone of critical thinking that allow for accurate diagnosis and early treatment.

There is one thing in medicine that has not changed over the millennia and that is the human body. Likewise, the most important instrument in medicine that a clinician uses on a daily basis is the human skill of critical thinking supported by our powerful sense of observation. It is important to understand this concept because it is central to the task of performing a comprehensive history and physical examination and, ultimately, culminating in an accurate diagnosis. This is true for any medical specialty, but particularly important for the specialty of rheumatology because rheumatic diseases are complex and can involve multiple organ systems.

There are more than 200 different rheumatic musculoskeletal diseases (RMDs) that affect both children and adults and their causes are just as diverse: immune system dysfunction, infection, inflammation, malignancy and deterioration over time. The European League Against Rheumatism and the American College of Rheumatology jointly agreed on terminology defining RMDs as a, "diverse group of diseases that commonly affect the joints but can affect any organ system of the body."[1,2] Most RMDs are chronic, systemic and can cause significant morbidity as well as early

MD Anderson Cancer Center, Galveston and League City, Unit: 1639, 2280 Gulf Freeway South, League City, TX 77573, USA
E-mail address: BASlusher@mdanderson.org

Physician Assist Clin 6 (2021) 15–22
https://doi.org/10.1016/j.cpha.2020.09.006
2405-7991/21/© 2020 Elsevier Inc. All rights reserved.

mortality, emphasizing the importance of early diagnosis and treatment. As such, rheumatology is considered a "cognitive specialty" requiring contemplation of the most common diagnoses while also considering rare conditions that may have similar presenting symptoms and physical examination findings (**Fig. 1**).

To facilitate accurate diagnostics and therapeutics, rheumatology health professionals must approach each patient encounter from the perspective of identifying patterns. Knowledge of the most common musculoskeletal conditions is essential so that review of systems questions and physical examination maneuvers can be narrowed from general to specific. Consider patterns consistent with the most common musculoskeletal conditions first to include mechanical low back pain, fractures, gout, fibromyalgia, injuries and overuse syndromes versus less common RMDs such as lupus, dermatomyositis or systemic sclerosis.

Although an accurate and early diagnosis is pivotal, many musculoskeletal complaints and conditions are self-limited and may only require symptomatic therapy. Others may take several visits and observation over time before clinical features necessary to establish a firm diagnosis are fully manifested.[3]

Identifying patterns begins with reviewing patient demographics such as age, sex, and ethnicity (**Table 1**). Age alone can build evidence in support of a particular diagnosis such as polymyalgia rheumatica or giant cell arteritis, both of which rarely occur in individuals younger than age 50 years old. Rheumatoid arthritis (RA) and systemic lupus erythematosus both have a propensity to affect women more frequently than men. In the case of systemic lupus erythematosus, it is more common and severe in Hispanic and African American women.

The cornerstone of evaluating patients with potential RMDs is a comprehensive history and physical examination with emphasis on features that may indicate inflammatory conditions. For asymmetric lower extremity joint dysfunction, consider gout osteoarthritis (OA) and reactive arthritis. For symmetric joint pain of the hands and wrists consider RA.

Identifying all the features of each symptom is fundamental to recognizing patterns of disease and to generating differential diagnoses.

SUBJECTIVE DATA: PATIENT PRESURVEY

Follow-up encounters of chronic conditions should include a review of the patient's self-management, response to treatment and functional capacity to include quality

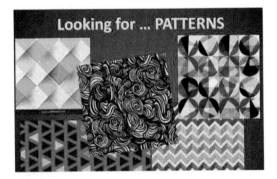

Fig. 1. Identifying patterns.

Table 1
Establishing patterns of RMDs based on associations with age, sex, and ethnicity

Parameter	Pattern A	Pattern B
Age	<50 y	>50 y
Potential RMD diagnosis	Repetitive strain, overuse syndromes, inflammatory bowel disease, reactive arthritis (associated with sexually transmitted infections)	Polymyalgia rheumatica, giant cell arteritis, osteoporotic fracture, pseudogout, malignancy
Sex	Male	Female
Potential RMD diagnosis	Reactive arthritis, Ankylosing spondylitis, Gout,	Systemic Lupus Erythematosus, Fibromyalgia, RA
Ethnicity	Caucasian	African American
Potential RMD diagnosis	Polymyalgia rheumatica, giant cell arteritis, osteoporotic fracture,	Systemic lupus erythematosus

of life. In preparing for the visit, review clinical records, the last note, and treatment plan. Consider the goal for the visit as well as what goals the patient may have. For clarity and transparency, specifically ask the patient what they would like to accomplish in the visit.

To gather the most data about the reason for the visit/history of present illness, use the OLD CARTS mnemonic (**Box 1**) to ensure completeness of the patient's report.

Information from OLD CARTS helps further delineate important patterns regarding 4 key features of musculoskeletal complaints:

1. Articular versus periarticular
2. Acute (<6 weeks) versus chronic (>6 weeks)
3. Inflammatory versus noninflammatory
4. Localized (monoarticular) versus diffuse (polyarticular)

Refer to **Table 2** for a helpful comparison of articular versus periarticular anatomy and associated physical examination findings.

Requesting patients to complete a previsit survey provides a wealth of information from the subjective patient-centered perspective that allows clinicians to begin organizing information. The survey can be short with just a few questions regarding interval history since last visit or longer with multiple questions requiring updates on new medicines, needed refills, side effects of medications, pain and fatigue ratings, etc. Patient

Box 1
Old carts mnemonic

Onset

Location

Duration

Character

Aggravate/alleviate

Radiate

Timing

Severity

Table 2
Comparison of articular versus periarticular anatomy and positive physical examination findings

Articular Anatomy	Periarticular Anatomy
Joint capsule, synovium, synovial fluid, cartilage, intra-articular ligaments and juxta-articular bone	Periarticular ligaments, tendons, bones, nerves, overlying skin, bursae, fascia and muscle
Physical examination findings	Physical examination findings
Swelling and tenderness of the entire joint, coarse crepitus, instability or locking deformity, decreased passive and active range of motion	Point or focal tenderness, decreased active range of motion, less commonly swelling

surveys can be integrated into electronic medical records as well to facilitate data transfer into the progress note. Review of systems can be gathered in the previsit survey as well. Patients can easily check off frequent symptoms they may be experiencing. These data must first be reviewed by the provider and then clarified in greater detail with the patient one on one.

An especially helpful tool for both provider and patient is the homunculus image with enlarged joints (**Fig. 2**). Patients can highlight or mark areas to identify the exact site of joint pain or dysfunction.

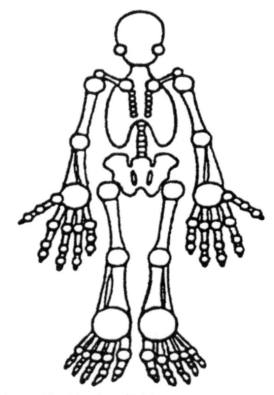

Fig. 2. Homunculus graphic with enlarged joints.

Providers can quickly get a visual to aid in pattern identification as well as planning to address issues during the visit. Consider the case of a patient that circles the entire homunculus indicating overall body pain. This may indicate a pattern of pain seen in the enthesopathy of psoriatic arthritis or the nociceptive pain of fibromyalgia syndrome.

PAST MEDICAL, FAMILY, AND SOCIAL HISTORY

Past medical, family, and social histories are necessary components of a comprehensive history and can have significant bearing on consideration of RMD diagnosis. A patient may report prior bouts of an eye condition requiring the use of steroid eye drops without knowing that this could indicate uveitis, an extra-articular manifestation of ankylosing spondylitis. How we frame our questions to the patient is important. For instance, asking a patient if they have a history of "uveitis" is not helpful because the general population is not familiar with this condition and may automatically respond "no" to the question. Instead, consider asking about prescription steroid use for eyes, skin, gastrointestinal, pulmonary, or other conditions. Family history is important, because a majority of RMDs have a genetic predisposition and overlap with other autoimmune conditions. Social history can uncover work related issues, such as chemical or toxic exposures or overuse syndromes.

Questioning regarding family history should not be restricted only to ascertaining whether other family members have a similar arthritis but should be as complete as possible regarding autoimmune diseases, many of which (e.g., RA, thyroid disease and diabetes) tend to cluster in families.[4,5]

REVIEW OF SYSTEMS

Owing to the systemic nature of RMDs, a thorough review of systems is necessary to establish possible involvement of other organ systems. As stated elsewhere in this article, a preliminary review of systems can be gathered in the patient's previsit survey and reviewed in greater detail during the encounter. Some organ systems are more frequently associated with particular RMDs and a constellation of symptoms can aid in diagnostic confirmation (**Table 3**).

For example, the pattern of lower extremity, monoarticular joint pain accompanied by urethritis can indicate reactive arthritis. Oligoarticular joint pain with skin rash and nail pitting can indicate psoriatic arthritis. In contrast, oligoarticular lower extremity joint pain with concomitant diarrhea can indicate spondyloarthropathy associated with inflammatory bowel disease.

Concerning inflammatory versus noninflammatory symptomatology, the following measures indicate an underlying inflammatory condition:

- Morning stiffness lasting more than 1 hour
- Significant fatigue
- Pain worsened by rest and improved with activity
- Systemic features (other organ system involvement)
- Positive response to corticosteroids

PATIENT INTERVIEW VISIT ENCOUNTER

Vital signs for patients with RMDs should include pain and fatigue ratings at each visit. Once treatment begins, these baseline indicators can demonstrate improvement in symptomatology and thus the effectiveness of treatment. Consider gait, motor

Table 3
Common systemic involvement associated with RMDs

Organ System	Feature	RMD Association
Skin	Malar rash	Systemic lupus erythematosus
	Scaly plaques with erythematous base, nail pitting	Psoriatic arthritis
	Heliotrope rash of the eyelid	Dermatomyositis
	Target lesion	Lyme arthritis
Eyes	Conjunctivitis	Reactive arthritis (Reiter syndrome – associated with urethritis, sexually transmitted infections)
	Uveitis	Bechet's disease, ankylosing spondylitis
Oral	Ulcerations	Systemic lupus erythematosus, RA, Bechet's disease
Lungs	Interstitial lung disease	Systemic sclerosis (scleroderma)
Gastrointestinal	Diarrhea	Inflammatory bowel disease
Genitourinary	Urethritis	Reactive arthritis (Reiter syndrome – associated with uveitis, sexually transmitted infections)

coordination, and posture both before and during the visit. Observe the patient walking into the examination room or getting up from the chair onto the examination table to document gait, motor activity, and general motor strength.

> Physical examination tip: Ask the patient to point to the site of pain using 1 finger. This technique aids in determining if pathology involves muscle, bone, or joint.

PHYSICAL EXAMINATION

Techniques of physical examination include inspection, palpation, and range of motion/maneuvers. There are 4 cardinal features of inflammation: swelling (tumor), redness (rubor), warmth (calor), and pain (dolor). On visual inspection, swelling, erythema and muscle atrophy can be noted. Swelling may not always be appreciated visually and generally requires confirmation by palpation of the joint and surrounding structures. Tenderness is determined by palpation—applying enough pressure over the joint so that the examiner's nail bed blanches. Tenderness can also be elicited by either passive or active range of motion and physical maneuvers.

Joint swelling can appear as bony swelling or synovial swelling. In the case of hand OA, bony swelling (bony hypertrophy) of the distal interphalangeal joints is bone hard on palpation, indicating bony overgrowth. In comparison, synovitis (synovial swelling) is the hallmark of RA and is squishy or spongy on palpation, indicating inflammation of the synovium. Swelling in the knee (knee effusion) is often appreciable on visual inspection and may be ballotable with palpation, that is, the bulge sign for small effusions and balloon sign for large effusions.

OA is asymmetric in presentation owing to underlying cause of overuse syndromes, degenerative wear and tear or history of injury or trauma. RA is strikingly symmetric in presentation owing to underlying cause of systemic inflammation often involving the small joints of bilateral hands, wrists, ankles and feet. For periarticular structures such as bursae, inflammation of the bursa (bursitis), is determined by tenderness on palpation over bony prominences.

> Physical examination tip: The metacarpophalangeal squeeze can be done bilaterally and is a quick way to assess tenderness in the hand.

For a complete joint examination, range of motion should include both passive and active range of motion. Active range of motion requires the patient to move the joint voluntarily. Passive range of motion, in contrast, is when the patient relaxes their limb and the examiner moves the joint through the full range of motion. Crepitus can be palpated or heard during range of motion testing and can be seen in both inflammatory and noninflammatory RMDs. In general, fine crepitus may be insignificant, whereas coarse crepitus may indicate long-standing joint dysfunction with bony remodeling. Bilateral muscle strength should be tested as well as significant muscle weakness may indicate more severe systemic involvement or inflammation (**Fig. 3**).

PUTTING IT ALL TOGETHER

The rheumatology health professional's most valuable tool for diagnosing and treating RMDs is the comprehensive history and physical examination. Review of system is the thread that links the subjective (patient-centered history) with the objective (provider-focused observation and physical examination). These 3 components are the cornerstone of critical thinking that allow for accurate diagnosis and early treatment.

Learning Objectives
1. Understand the importance of history, review of systems and physical examination as the cornerstone of accurate diagnosis and treatment of RMDs.
2. Identify components of the comprehensive medical, family, and social histories of a patient presenting with RMDs that may indicate a pattern of inflammation.
3. Understand the link between subjective (patient history) and review of systems to the objective (physical examination) that is, the basis for pattern identification in RMDs.
4. Recall important characteristics of physical examination that determines inflammatory versus noninflammatory conditions.

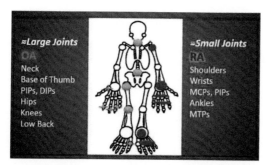

Fig. 3. Small joints (*in red*) are more often affected by RA: metacarpophalangeal and proximal interphalangeal joints of the hands, wrists, shoulders, ankles, and metatarsophalangeal joints. Large joints or joints involved in repetitive range of motion (*in blue*) are commonly affected by OA, namely, the knee, hip, lumbar spine, cervical spine, distal interphalangeal joints, and carpometacarpal joint.

REFERENCES

1. van der Heijde D, Daikh DI, Betteridge N, et al. Common language description of the term rheumatic and musculoskeletal diseases (RMD s) for use in communication with the lay public, healthcare providers, and other stakeholders endorsed by the European League Against Rheumatism (EULAR) and the American College of Rheumatology (ACR). Arthritis Rheumatol 2018;70:826–31.
2. West SG, Kolfenback J, editors. Rheumatology secrets. 4th edition. Philadelphia: Elsevier; 2020.
3. Cush JJ, Kavanaugh AF, Stein CM. Rheumatology: diagnosis and therapeutics. 2nd edition. Philadelphia: Lippincott, Williams & Wilkins; 2004.
4. Klippel JH, Stone JH, Crofford LJ, et al, editors. Primer on the rheumatic diseases. 13th edition. New York: Springer Science+Business Media, LLC; 2008.
5. Bickley LS, editor. Bates' guide to physical examination and history taking. 12th edition. Philadelphia,: Wolters Kluwer; 2017.

Osteoarthritis and Its Management

What the Physician Assistant Needs to Know

Katie F. Huffman, MA[a],*, Tina H. Thornhill, PharmD, BCGP[b],
Kirsten R. Ambrose, MS, CCRC[a], Amanda E. Nelson, MD, MSCR[a,c],
Leigh F. Callahan, PhD[a,c,d,e,f]

KEYWORDS

- Osteoarthritis • Public health • Treatment • Prevention

KEY POINTS

- Affecting over 32 million US adults, osteoarthritis (OA) is the most common form of arthritis and results in considerable personal and economic burden.
- Increased rates of comorbidities, reduced levels of physical activity, and the potential for adverse effects of medications contribute to increased risk of mortality among patients with OA.
- The most effective treatment and prevention strategies for OA include physical activity, weight management, self-management education, and injury prevention.

INTRODUCTION

Osteoarthritis (OA) is a complex disease that warrants particular clinical attention given its extensive patient and economic burden, combined with its connection to other chronic conditions and the fact that there is currently no cure.[1,2] Characterized by joint pain and stiffness, and most commonly found in the knees, hips, hands, feet, and spine, OA can have a profound impact on patients' quality of life (QOL) and daily activities.[2] Further, evidence supports the role of OA in an increased risk of

[a] Osteoarthritis Action Alliance, Thurston Arthritis Research Center, University of North Carolina at Chapel Hill, 3300 Thurston Building, CB 7280, Chapel Hill, NC 27599-7280, USA; [b] Campbell University College of Pharmacy & Health Sciences, P.O. Box 1090, 234 J.P. Riddle Building, Buies Creek, NC 27506, USA; [c] Department of Medicine, University of North Carolina; [d] Department of Orthopaedics, University of North Carolina; [e] Department of Social Medicine, University of North Carolina; [f] Department of Epidemiology, Gillings School of Global Public Health, University of North Carolina
* Corresponding author. Thurston Arthritis Research Center, University of North Carolina at Chapel Hill, 3300 Thurston Building, CB 7280, Chapel Hill, NC 27599-7280.
E-mail address: Katie_huffman@med.unc.edu

Physician Assist Clin 6 (2021) 23–40
https://doi.org/10.1016/j.cpha.2020.08.003
2405-7991/21/© 2020 Elsevier Inc. All rights reserved.
physicianassistant.theclinics.com

premature mortality; thus OA should be understood and treated as a serious disease.[1,3] The most effective management and prevention strategies for OA require a partnership between providers and patients, pairing clinical care with patient self-management activities such as physical activity, weight loss, education, and injury prevention.[4]

EPIDEMIOLOGY
Prevalence

OA is a serious disease[1] and is increasing in prevalence, resulting in enormous socioeconomic costs for individuals and society as a whole.[2] The US Centers for Disease Control and Prevention (CDC) estimate that 1 in 4 (or 54.4 million) US adults have some form of arthritis, a figure that is projected to reach 78 million by 2040.[5] Of the over 100 types of arthritis, OA is by far the most common, affecting an estimated 32.5 million US adults.[2] Not only is prevalence of OA increasing, but patient characteristics are changing, in part because of rising rates of obesity, physical inactivity, and joint injury among young people.[6]

Personal and Economic Burden of Osteoarthritis

The personal toll of OA is notable (**Fig. 1**). In fact, the burden of OA has been compared with that of rheumatoid arthritis, a multisystem autoimmune disease known to have severe patient consequences.[6–9] People with OA experience greater levels of pain, fatigue, disability, and functional limitations than people without.[1] Although OA pain varies by patient, severe joint pain is not uncommon. Approximately one-fourth of adults with arthritis experience severe joint pain with a score of 7 or greater on a 0 to 10 pain scale in the previous 30 days.[10]

Chronic and acute pain from OA can result in depression and other mood disturbances, functional disabilities, and work limitations. Musculoskeletal disorders are one of the greatest contributors to years lived with disability, with OA following back and neck pain in that category.[11] Almost 44% of people with arthritis have arthritis-attributable activity limitations, defined by the CDC as self-reported limitations in usual activities because of arthritis symptoms,[5] and by 2040, an estimated 11% of all adults will experience arthritis-attributable activity limitations.[12]

In addition to the burden of disease on patients' QOL, OA is expensive for individuals and the economy. The overall economic burden associated with OA in the United States is estimated at $136.8 billion annually, which includes both direct medical costs and indirect costs.[2] Annual direct medical costs reach $65 billion,[2] while indirect costs are estimated at greater than $71 billion.[2] Indirect costs include increased rates of absenteeism, with workers with OA missing an average of 2 more days per year than workers without OA. Presenteeism, or reduced productivity while on the job, is difficult to calculate but is no doubt costly for businesses.[13]

Comorbidities and Mortality

Patients with OA often have additional chronic conditions that can significantly impact disease progression and management. Most people with OA have at least 1 additional comorbid condition, while about one-third have 5 or more chronic conditions.[1] Patients with diabetes and/or heart disease are more likely to have arthritis than the general population; in fact, almost half of those with heart disease (49%) or diabetes (47%), and nearly one-third of those with obesity (31%) also have arthritis.[5] Depression and anxiety are also reported by about one-third of individuals with arthritis.[14,15]

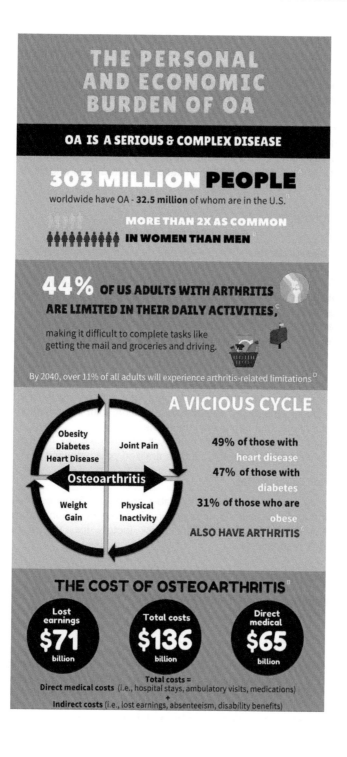

THE PERSONAL AND ECONOMIC BURDEN OF OA

OA IS A SERIOUS & COMPLEX DISEASE

303 MILLION PEOPLE

worldwide have OA - **32.5 million** of whom are in the U.S.

MORE THAN 2X AS COMMON IN WOMEN THAN MEN

44% OF US ADULTS WITH ARTHRITIS ARE LIMITED IN THEIR DAILY ACTIVITIES,

making it difficult to complete tasks like getting the mail and groceries and driving.

By 2040, over 11% of all adults will experience arthritis-related limitations

A VICIOUS CYCLE

Obesity
Diabetes
Heart Disease

Joint Pain

Osteoarthritis

Weight Gain

Physical Inactivity

49% of those with heart disease
47% of those with diabetes
31% of those who are obese
ALSO HAVE ARTHRITIS

THE COST OF OSTEOARTHRITIS

Lost earnings
$71 billion

Total costs
$136 billion

Direct medical
$65 billion

Total costs =
Direct medical costs (i.e., hospital stays, ambulatory visits, medications)
+
Indirect costs (i.e., lost earnings, absenteeism, disability benefits)

Comorbid conditions can impact providers' ability to detect the presence of OA and to tailor appropriate management strategies. When combined with arthritis, comorbidities contribute to a vicious cycle of pain, disability, obesity, and inactivity. Patients with OA may find it more difficult to engage in physical activity—a treatment option for many chronic conditions, including OA—which can lead to extra body weight, increased heart disease, and/or diabetes symptoms, worse joint pain, and less movement. (see **Fig. 1**). Additionally, comorbid conditions can complicate medication selection for treating OA symptoms.

Knee and hip OA have been linked to higher rates of mortality.[1,11,16,17] Increased rates of mortality among people with OA are likely caused by other comorbidities, decreased physical activity, mobility limitations, and adverse effects of medication in addition to the disease pathology itself.[1]

PATHOPHYSIOLOGY
Pathogenesis

OA has long been understood from a wear and tear or mechanical perspective as cartilage and synovial fluid degrade in commonly affected joints (eg, hands, hips, knees, or spine), leading to pain, stiffness, and reduced joint function.[18] However, OA is far more complex than a mechanical breakdown of joint tissues and should not be referred to as simply degenerative joint disease (**Fig. 2**). This complexity is reflected in the Osteoarthritis Research Society International's comprehensive definition of OA:

"a disorder involving movable joints characterized by cell stress and extracellular matrix degradation initiated by micro- and macro-injury that activates maladaptive repair responses including pro-inflammatory pathways of innate immunity. The disease manifests first as a molecular derangement (abnormal joint tissue metabolism) followed by anatomic, and/or physiologic derangements (characterized by cartilage degradation, bone remodeling, osteophyte formation, joint inflammation and loss of normal joint function), that can culminate in illness."[19]

Pain associated with OA is likely the result of this complex interplay of factors including mechanical, inflammatory, and centralized pain pathways.[20]

Risk Factors for Osteoarthritis

Categorizing risk factors for OA as modifiable or nonmodifiable can help providers detect OA and assist patients in engaging in effective prevention and management strategies. Nonmodifiable and modifiable risk factors for OA are described in **Tables 1** and **2**, respectively.

CLINICAL PRESENTATION AND DIAGNOSIS

OA can best be diagnosed through a combination of assessments: patient history and symptoms, physical examination, and imaging.

Fig. 1. The personal and economic burden of osteoarthritis. [a]Kloppenburg M, Berenbaum F. Osteoarthritis year in review 2019: epidemiology and therapy. Osteoarthritis Cartilage. 2020. [b]United States Bone and Joint Initiative. The burden of musculoskeletal diseases in the United States (BMUS). In: Fourth ed. Rosemont, IL. 2018: Available at https://www.boneandjointburden.org/fourth-edition. Accessed January 17,2020. [c]Barbour KE, Helmick CG, Boring M, Brady TJ. Vital signs: prevalence of doctor-diagnosed arthritis and arthritis-attributable activity limitation - United States, 2013-2015. MMWR Morb Mortal Wkly Rep 2017;66(9):246-253. [d]Hootman JM, Helmick CG, Barbour KE, et al. Updated projected prevalence of self-reported doctor-diagnosed arthritis and arthritis-attributable activity limitation among US Adults, 2015-2040. Arthritis Rheumatol 2016;68(7):1582-1587.

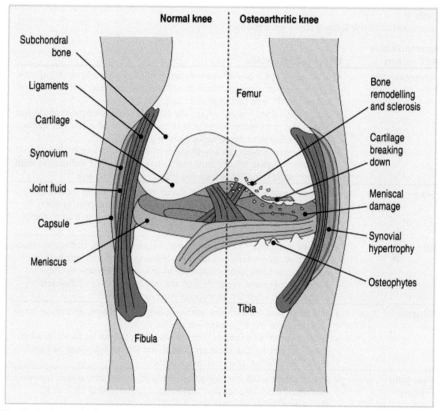

Fig. 2. Pathogenic features consistent with OA. *From* Hunter DJ, Felson DT. Osteoarthritis. BMJ. 2006;332(7542): 639-642, reprinted with permission..

Patient History and Symptoms

OA symptoms vary depending on the affected joint and the severity of disease. Common symptoms patients may describe include:

- Pain that is relieved by rest and aggravated by too little or too much activity
- Increasing pain as the day goes on
- Stiffness that is worse after prolonged inactivity and that is reduced after some movement
- Crackling or grinding noises during flexing of the joint
- Mild swelling around the joint

Patients also might describe functional limitations or difficulty performing daily routines.[42] Everyday activities like dressing, bathing, cooking, writing, climbing stairs, and driving, as well as social activities such as visiting with friends and relatives and being involved in the community may be impacted by OA.[43]

Hawker and colleagues[44] described 3 stages of OA relative to patients' experience with pain and functional limitations (**Box 1**). Patients may also report sleep disturbances characteristic of insomnia (inadequate sleep, difficulty initiating or maintaining sleep and/or feeling unrefreshed after sleeping). The prevalence of sleep disturbance among people with knee OA is estimated at more than 70%.[45]

Table 1 Nonmodifiable risk factors for osteoarthritis	
Nonmodifiable Risk Factors	**Evidence and Details**
Advancing age	• Advancing age is one of the greatest risk factors for OA, resulting from age-related changes in muscle function, joint position and movement, tissue health, and cartilage structure.[18,21] • Aging itself does not automatically lead to the development of OA but makes the joint more vulnerable in the presence of other risk factors and contributes to more rapid disease progression.[21] • 88% of people with OA are 45 years of age or older, and 43% are 65 years of age or older.[2] However, more than half of individuals with symptomatic knee OA are younger than 65 years of age.[22]
Sex	• 62% of people with OA are women,[2] although among individuals younger than 45 years of age, OA is more common among men.[22] • Females have an increased risk of OA, especially in the hands, feet, and knees.[22]
Ethnicity	• 78% of individuals with OA are non-Hispanic whites, but within their respective race/ethnic groups, non-Hispanic black and Hispanic populations have higher rates of OA than non-Hispanic whites.[2] • African-Americans, regardless of sex, are more likely to develop symptomatic knee OA compared with other races.[23]
Genetics	• Multiple gene interactions within collagen, cartilage, and bone may contribute to the development of OA. • According to twin studies, risk of inheriting OA varies by joint, with spine OA having the greatest heritability (70%), followed by hand (65%), hip (60%), and then knee (40%).[24]
Prior joint injury	• Post-traumatic OA involving the cartilage, ligaments, and/or meniscus can result from injuries and makes up approximately 12% of all OA cases.[25] • Someone who has had a torn anterior cruciate ligament (ACL) or meniscus is more than twice as likely to develop knee OA and 4 times more likely to undergo an eventual total knee replacement.[20,23,26] • 10%–90% of young athletes with an ACL injury will develop OA within 10 to 20 years of the injury.[27] • Unfortunately, surgical reconstruction and rehabilitation do not appear to mitigate the risk of developing OA following these types of injuries.[27]

Physical Examination and Associated Examinations

The affected joint(s) may show signs of tenderness or mild swelling. Joints with OA are not usually warm, red, or markedly swollen. Crepitus, reduced muscle mass (eg, of quadriceps or thenar muscles) or joint deformity (caused by bony enlargement, ankylosis, or malalignment) may also be noticeable. Osteophytes may result in visible deformities—especially in the distal interphalangeal and proximal interphalangeal joints in the hands—and can restrict range of motion.[46] Heberden and/or Bouchard nodes are sometimes present in hand OA; these are bony enlargements of the distal or proximal interphalangeal joints, respectively.[47] Observing a patient's gait in the clinic may help detect an uneven or unstable gait indicative of knee or hip OA and can reveal knee malalignment.[39]

Imaging

Imaging is generally not needed to guide treatment decisions, but in rare cases, radiographs may be used to confirm the diagnosis or to rule out other potential diagnoses

Table 2
Modifiable risk factors for osteoarthritis

Modifiable Risk Factors	Evidence and Details

Excess weight	• The most significant modifiable risk factor for the development of OA of the knee is obesity.
	• Obesity is associated with higher rates of disability among people with arthritis.[28,29]
	• Ten pounds of additional weight increases the force exerted on the knee by up to 60 pounds with each step.[30]
	• For each kilogram (2.2 pounds) of excess weight, the risk of developing OA increases by approximately 10%.[28]
	• Both mechanical and metabolic aspects of obesity contribute to the development of OA.
	  ○ Obesity affects gait mechanics and distribution of weight across the affected and nonaffected joints, resulting in tissue or cartilage damage.[31,32]
	  ○ Excess body weight has been associated with increased risk of hand OA,[33] and metabolic syndrome is more prevalent in people with OA than those without.[33,34]
	  ○ The metabolic pathologic changes that occur in a joint with OA have been directly linked to insulin resistance, low bone density, alterations in collagen production and the impact of LDL oxidation on bone formation, and development of low-grade synovial inflammation.[35]

Occupation and sports	• Certain occupations involving prolonged standing, squatting, lifting, kneeling, and repetitive motion that results in excessive mechanical stress on a joint increase the risk of OA and can worsen symptoms.[36,37] • In addition to elite-level athletes (soccer, long-distance running, weight lifting and wrestling), nonelite soccer athletes have also been found at risk of developing OA.[38]
Avoiding joint injury	• Although injuries from occupational activities, sports, or accidental falls may not be entirely preventable, steps can be taken to reduce their incidence or impact in later life. • Injury prevention programs that include stretching, strengthening, and neuromuscular training components have been shown to reduce ACL injuries in athletes by over 50%.[27]
Joint position and muscle strength	• Knees that are mechanically misaligned- resulting in either varus or valgus alignments- can result in increased risk of knee OA.[39] • Weaker quadriceps strength is associated with increased functional disability and pain in people with knee OA.[40,41]

(eg, osteonecrosis, fracture, other types of arthritis). Radiographs are the most common, cost-effective, and accessible form of imaging for OA. Radiographs can reveal important characteristics of OA such as osteophytes, joint space narrowing, subchondral cysts, and sclerosis and joint malalignment or deformity (**Fig. 3**). Patients with radiographic OA may not suffer from OA symptoms, while other patients may experience OA symptoms before the disease is detected on examination or radiograph.[48,49] Patients' experiences with OA pain and functional limitations are the more important indicators for providers to use in diagnosing and managing OA.[48]

OSTEOARTHRITIS MANAGEMENT

Management strategies span an array of therapies such as physical activity, weight management, injury prevention and education; pharmacologic therapies such as

> **Box 1**
> **Stages of osteoarthritis based on patient experience[44]**
>
> - Early OA: pain is infrequent and predictable and is brought on by specific movements or activities; patients continue to have well-preserved joint function and QOL
>
> - Mid-OA: pain is predictable but more constant; there is an increased presence of unpredictable symptoms such as locking, and patients experience some impairment of function, participation in activities, and QOL
>
> - Advanced OA: pain is described as persistent, dull, and aching with intermittent episodes of unpredictable sharp pain; patients commonly experience fatigue and impaired function and are significantly restricted in activities and QOL

oral or topical nonsteroidal anti-inflammatory drugs (NSAIDs) and joint injections; and/or surgical interventions.[4,50] Although there are many national and international organizations that release guidelines on the management of OA, the following recommendations adhere to the 2019 guidelines from the American College of Rheumatology (ACR) on the management of knee, hip, and hand OA.[4]

The recommendations fall broadly into 2 categories—physical/behavioral and pharmacologic—which should be used concurrently as well as tailored to each patient based on his or her medical history, personal preferences, coexisting health conditions, and current medication regimen.

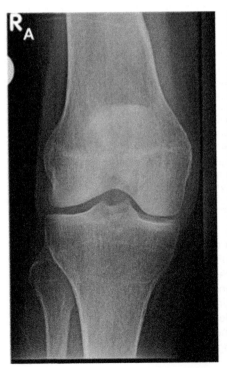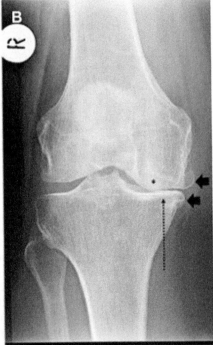

Fig. 3. Radiograph images of knee with OA. (*A*). Right knee with normal joint space, no osteophytes. (*B*). Right knee with sclerosis (*), medial joint space narrowing (*long dashed arrow*), osteophytes (*black arrows*). (*Courtesy of* AE. Nelson Johnston, MD, County Osteoarthritis Project.)

Educational, Behavioral, Psychosocial, and Physical Management

An extensive range of educational, behavioral, psychosocial, and physical interventions for OA exists, and thus will be categorized by referrals to other specialties, self-management strategies, and assistive devices. A more thorough list of modalities and explanation of evidence behind them can be found in the 2019 ACR Guideline (**Table 3**).[4]

Referrals to other specialties

Physical and occupational therapy Physical and occupational therapists can play a central role in the care of patients with OA throughout the disease course.[4] Not only will these professionals assist when patients experience functional limitations,[51] but they can also connect individuals to many other effective OA interventions such as exercise and self-management programs, home adaptations, and appropriate use of assistive devices.[4]

Mental health provider Individuals with OA are more likely to experience anxiety and depression compared to those without.[52] A patient's mental health can interfere with his or her QOL, daily activities, and ability to engage in effective OA management

Table 3
Recommendations for physical, psychosocial, and mind-body approaches for the management of osteoarthritis of the hand, knee, and hip

Intervention	Joint		
	Hand	Knee	Hip
Exercise			
Balance training			
Weight loss			
Self-efficacy and self-management programs			
Tai chi			
Yoga			
Cognitive behavioral therapy			
Cane			
Tibiofemoral knee braces		(Tibiofemoral)	
Patellofemoral braces		(Patellofemoral)	
Kinesiotaping	(First carpometacarpal)		
Hand orthosis	(First carpometacarpal)		
Hand orthosis	(other joints)		
Modified shoes			
Lateral and medial wedged insoles			
Acupuncture			
Thermal interventions			
Paraffin			
Radiofrequency ablation			
Massage therapy			
Manual therapy with/without exercise			
Iontophoresis	(First carpometacarpal)		
Pulsed vibration therapy			
Transcutaneous electrical nerve stimulation			

Strongly recommended
Conditionally recommended
Strongly recommended against
Conditionally recommended against
No recommendation

From Kolasinski SL, Neogi T, Hochberg MC, et al. 2019 American College of Rheumatology/Arthritis Foundation Guideline for the Management of Osteoarthritis of the Hand, Hip, and Knee. Arthritis Rheumatol. 2020;72:220-233; with permission.

strategies.[53] Referral to a mental health provider for cognitive behavioral therapy may help with a patient's ability to cope with OA symptoms such as pain, changes in sleep and mood, and functional limitations.

Rheumatology A referral to rheumatology may be indicated for evaluation of other etiologies if initial attempts at treatment are ineffective or there are signs of more inflammatory features.

Sports medicine Sports medicine providers work with athletes, teams, and individuals, focusing on injury prevention and nonoperative treatments following sports injuries.[54] They can recommend exercise, strength conditioning, and injury prevention programs and may be able to administer or advise on intra-articular injections.

Orthopedics For patients with more severe OA and associated disability and for whom more conservative treatments have failed, consideration of intra-articular injections or surgery may be needed.[51] In lower extremity OA, surgical interventions that are most commonly recommended include partial/total joint replacement and osteotomy.[51,55] Total joint replacement can greatly improve QOL for patients with OA. However, joint replacements are not without risk, and up to 20% of patients who have this surgery continue to experience chronic pain, particularly those with presurgical conditions of widespread pain, high-intensity pain, complex comorbidities, and mental illness.[56]

Self-management strategies
Physical activity Exercise is the most universally recommended intervention for management of OA in all joints.[4,50,55] Although no standard exercise prescription has been established, improvements in pain and function have been confirmed from walking, cycling, aquatic activities, resistance training, and stretching (**Box 2**). Given that the best exercise program is the one that a patient will begin and sustain, patient preference should be central in regard to type, location, frequency, intensity, and duration.[4]

Weight loss Even small amounts of weight loss can help patients achieve improved pain and function, particularly in knee and hip OA. In the IDEA trial (Intensive Diet and Exercise for Arthritis), not only did patients with knee OA who were overweight experience a 50% reduction in pain scores after losing a modest amount of weight (10% of body weight), but there were also benefits to joint load and inflammation.[51,63] Weight loss is best combined with physical activity to optimize benefits to OA symptoms.[4]

Self-efficacy and education Self-management education (SME) programs educate and empower people with chronic diseases to understand their disease and manage its impact on their daily life. Participants in SME programs can experience improvements in self-confidence, self-rated health, exercise levels, and mental health.[64] Examples of appropriate programs for people with OA include the Arthritis Self-Management Program (online) and Chronic Disease Self-Management Program (online or in person).[65]

Assistive devices
Braces are recommended for use in patients with knee OA to improve walking ability and joint stability and to reduce pain. In knee and hand OA, kinesiotaping may be beneficial. For hand OA, splints or other orthoses and gloves or paraffin can be used for support and pain relief. Modified shoes and insoles have not shown clear benefits and are therefore not recommended. Canes are strongly recommended for patients with knee and hip OA when ambulation or balance is impaired. Guidance on selection, fitting, and use of all of these devices is best left to a specialist.[4]

Box 2
Physical activity for patients with osteoarthritis

Physical activity recommendations
The National Physical Activity Guidelines recommend that adults engage in 150 minutes per week of moderate intensity aerobic exercise, combined with 2 days of strengthening activities.[57] However, it is possible that as little as 45 minutes of moderate-to-vigorous activity per week could help patients with lower extremity OA improve or maintain their function.[58] Patients in pain may be hesitant to participate in exercise given that initially, movement can increase pain; for some individuals, referral to a supervised physical activity program, physical therapist, or fitness professional could be beneficial.[4] Balance exercises and mind-body practices such as tai chi and yoga are also recommended forms of physical activity for people with knee and hip OA.[4]

Evidence-based physical activity programs
There are several evidence-based physical activity programs designed specifically for or proven to benefit people with OA.
Offered in community settings (eg, senior center, YMCA), these programs are facilitated by trained leaders and help participants of all fitness levels engage in various types of exercise using safe and sustainable strategies. Examples include:
- Active Living Every Day[59]
- Fit and Strong![60]
- Walk With Ease[61]
- Enhance Fitness.[62]

More information about these programs and how to locate course offerings in a specific location can be found at https://oaaction.unc.edu/RxLinks.

Pharmacologic Management

Because no disease-modifying therapies have been identified for OA, pharmacologic interventions are used to help improve patients' pain, mobility, and function (**Table 4**). It is important to educate patients that these medications are for symptomatic relief and do not affect the underlying disease process.

Oral analgesics

Oral nonsteroidal anti-inflammatory drugs (NSAIDs) are strongly recommended in the treatment of knee, hip, and hand OA. The ACR does not recommend one particular NSAID over another; trials of different NSAIDs may be considered to determine the most effective medication for a given patient. NSAIDs carry a black box warning for their gastrointestinal (eg, ulcers and bleeds) and cardiovascular (eg, hypertension, heart failure, stroke, and myocardial infarction) risks. NSAIDs can also cause renal adverse effects including acute renal failure. Because of these possible adverse drug reactions, caution should be used when prescribing NSAIDs, emphasizing the lowest effective dose for the shortest period possible. Comorbid conditions should be carefully considered before considering NSAID therapy.

Other oral analgesics conditionally recommended by ACR include acetaminophen, duloxetine, and tramadol.[4] Acetaminophen, a simple analgesic, has fewer adverse effects than oral NSAIDs and may be a safer alternative when patients are not candidates for NSAID therapy, although it may be less effective. Nontramadol opioids have only shown modest improvements in pain, and given their well-established risks, should be avoided if possible.

Topical analgesics

Topical NSAIDs may be preferred over oral analgesics given their reduced systemic exposure. They are most effective for superficial joints such as the knee and hand. Topical NSAIDs also carry a black box warning and should be prescribed with caution

Table 4
Recommendations for the pharmacologic management of osteoarthritis of the hand, knee, and hip

Intervention	Joint		
	Hand	Knee	Hip
Topical nonsteroidal anti-inflammatory drugs			
Topical capsaicin			
Oral nonsteroidal anti-inflammatory drugs			
Intraarticular glucocorticoid injection			
Ultrasound-guided intraarticular glucocorticoid injection			
Intraarticular glucocorticoid injection compared to other injections			
Acetaminophen			
Duloxetine			
Tramadol			
Non-tramadol opioids			
Colchicine			
Fish oil			
Vitamin D			
Bisphosphonates			
Glucosamine			
Chondroitin sulfate			
Hydroxychloroquine			
Methotrexate			
Intraarticular hyaluronic acid injection	(First carpometacarpal)		
Intraarticular botulinum toxin			
Prolotherapy			
Platelet-rich plasma			
Stem cell injection			
Biologics (tumor necrosis factor inhibitors, interleukin-1 receptor antagonists)			

Strongly recommended
Conditionally recommended
Strongly recommended against
Conditionally recommended against
No recommendation

From Kolasinski SL, Neogi T, Hochberg MC, et al. 2019 American College of Rheumatology/Arthritis Foundation Guideline for the Management of Osteoarthritis of the Hand, Hip, and Knee. Arthritis Rheumatol. 2020;72:220-233; with permission.

in older adults and patients with more comorbid conditions, but they are often more appropriate for use than oral NSAIDs.[4]

Topical capsaicin (available without a prescription) can be used for knee OA with small effect but has not been shown to be especially effective in hand or hip OA. Not enough evidence is currently available to make a recommendation about the use of topical lidocaine.[4]

Injections
Intra-articular glucocorticoids are recommended for the treatment of knee, hip, and hand OA, although effects are short-term. Other types of intra-articular injections such as hyaluronans, platelet-rich plasma and stem cells, are not recommended because of lack of evidence.[4] Patients should discuss the use of injections with a qualified provider.

OSTEOARTHRITIS PREVENTION

Given the extensive patient and economic burden and the rising prevalence of OA, it is important to recognize cases in clinical care where prevention strategies can be implemented to prevent the onset of OA or to slow its progression. Current evidence-based prevention strategies fall largely into 2 categories: weight management and injury prevention.

Weight Management

Being overweight or obese is implicated as a risk factor for many chronic conditions including diabetes, heart disease, cancer, and premature death.[66] Patients of all age groups who are overweight would benefit from counseling about the importance of achieving and maintaining a healthy weight to combat these diseases.[67] Preserving joint health and function should be another compelling reason to manage weight. Not only are individuals who are overweight at greater risk of developing OA, but they are more likely to experience disability once they have OA.[28,29]

Injury Prevention

Although injuries sustained through sports, on the job, or from accidents are not always avoidable, policies and practices can be implemented in occupational[68] and athletic settings[27] to reduce the risk of joint injuries. Participating in a neuromuscular training program can reduce athletes' risk of knee injury by over 50%.[27] Effective injury prevention programs include stretching, strengthening, and plyometric and balance exercises and can be implemented in as little as 15 minutes 2 to 3 times per week.[69] Injury prevention is especially important for people who have previously sustained an injury[70,71] and for those individuals who are overweight yet who are also physically active[72,73]; both groups are at greater risk of injury.[70–73]

Patients with OA are not only more likely to experience falls but are also more likely to sustain a fracture from a fall than those without OA. Patients at risk of falling should be counseled to engage in or increase their physical activity to build strength and improve balance to reduce their risk of fall-related injuries.[74]

SUMMARY

Given today's brief clinic visits combined with the competing demands of managing multiple comorbidities like diabetes, hypertension, and heart disease, OA can be overlooked or minimized by both the patient and provider. However, when viewed within the context of a patient's ability to manage his or her other chronic conditions and overall QOL, OA plays a critical role in patient care. An individualized and multimodal treatment strategy for OA will not only contribute to prolonged mobility and reduced pain and stiffness but also has the potential to positively impact management of patients' other chronic conditions and improve QOL.

CLINICS CARE POINTS

- Detection of the signs and symptoms of OA, particularly early in the disease process, can better equip Physician Assistants and their patients in selecting the most appropriate management pathway for both the OA symptoms and other comorbid conditions.
- A vicious cycle of OA, pain, disability, obesity, and comorbidities can significantly impact OA disease progression and management as well as the treatment of other conditions.
- The most effective approach to managing patients' OA symptoms or delaying the progression of OA is through the use of educational, behavioral, psychosocial and physical interventions.

- Every patient with OA is different and will require a tailored treatment approach comprised of multi-modal and personalized recommendations.
- The Arthritis Foundation's Walk With Ease is just one example of an evidence-based physical activity program proven to benefit people with OA and can be easily accessed in many communities or online.

ACKNOWLEDGMENTS

The Osteoarthritis Action Alliance (OAAA) is a national public health coalition committed to increasing awareness about OA, promoting evidence-based interventions for OA, and providing resources for public and professional education in support of OA prevention and management. More information and resources for providers and patients are available on the OAAA website (http://oaaction.unc.edu/) and toolkit for primary care providers (https://oaaction.unc.edu/resource-library/modules/).

FUNDING:

This publication was supported by Cooperative Agreement Number, 6 NU58DP006262-04-01, funded by the CDC. Its contents are solely the responsibility of the authors and do not necessarily represent the official views of the CDC or the US Department of Health and Human Services.

DISCLOSURE

The authors have nothing to disclose.

REFERENCES

1. Osteoarthritis Research Society International. Osteoarthritis: a serious disease, submitted to the U.S. food and drug administration. 2016. Available at: https://www.oarsi.org/sites/default/files/docs/2016/oarsi_white_paper_oa_serious_disease_121416_1.pdf. Accessed January 16, 2020.
2. United States Bone and Joint Initiative: The Burden of Musculoskeletal Diseases in the United States (BMUS). 3rd Edition. Rosemont (IL): USBJI. Available at https://www.boneandjointburden.org/third-edition/right. Accessed January 17, 2020.
3. Cleveland RJ, Nelson AE, Callahan LF. Knee and hip osteoarthritis as predictors of premature death: a review of the evidence. Clin Exp Rheumatol 2019;37:24–30. Suppl 120(5.
4. Kolasinski SL, Neogi T, Hochberg MC, et al. 2019 American college of rheumatology/Arthritis foundation guideline for the management of osteoarthritis of the hand, hip, and knee. Arthritis Rheum 2020;72:220–33.
5. Barbour KE, Helmick CG, Boring M, et al. Vital signs: prevalence of doctor-diagnosed arthritis and arthritis-attributable activity limitation - United States, 2013-2015. MMWR Morb Mortal Wkly Rep 2017;66(9):246–53.
6. Hawker GA. Osteoarthritis is a serious disease. Clin Exp Rheumatol 2019;37:3–6. Suppl 120(5).
7. El-Haddad C, Castrejon I, Gibson KA, et al. MDHAQ/RAPID3 scores in patients with osteoarthritis are similar to or higher than in patients with rheumatoid arthritis: a cross-sectional study from current routine rheumatology care at four sites. RMD Open 2017;3(1):e000391.
8. Chua JR, Jamal S, Riad M, et al. Disease burden in osteoarthritis is similar to that of rheumatoid arthritis at initial rheumatology visit and significantly greater six months later. Arthritis Rheumatol 2019;71(8):1276–84.

9. Pincus T, Castrejon I, Yazici Y, et al. Osteoarthritis is as severe as rheumatoid arthritis: evidence over 40 years according to the same measure in each disease. Clin Exp Rheumatol 2019;37:7–17. Suppl 120(5).

10. Barbour KE, Boring M, Helmick CG, et al. Prevalence of severe joint pain among adults with doctor-diagnosed arthritis - United States, 2002-2014. MMWR Morb Mortal Wkly Rep 2016;65(39):1052–6.

11. Kloppenburg M, Berenbaum F. Osteoarthritis year in review 2019: epidemiology and therapy. Osteoarthritis Cartilage 2020;28(3):242–8.

12. Hootman JM, Helmick CG, Barbour KE, et al. Updated projected prevalence of self-reported doctor-diagnosed arthritis and arthritis-attributable activity limitation among US adults, 2015-2040. Arthritis Rheum 2016;68(7):1582–7.

13. Menon J. Osteoarthritis related absenteeism and activity limitations. Osteoarthritis Cartilage 2015;23:A343.

14. Murphy LB, Sacks JJ, Brady TJ, et al. Anxiety and depression among US adults with arthritis: prevalence and correlates. Arthritis Care Res (Hoboken) 2012;64(7): 968–76.

15. Guglielmo D, Hootman JM, Boring MA, et al. Symptoms of anxiety and depression among adults with arthritis - United States, 2015-2017. MMWR Morb Mortal Wkly Rep 2018;67(39):1081–7.

16. Cleveland RJ, Alvarez C, Schwartz TA, et al. The impact of painful knee osteoarthritis on mortality: a community-based cohort study with over 24 years of follow-up. Osteoarthritis Cartilage 2019;27(4):593–602.

17. Nuesch E, Dieppe P, Reichenbach S, et al. All cause and disease specific mortality in patients with knee or hip osteoarthritis: population based cohort study. BMJ 2011;342:d1165.

18. Loeser R. Pathogenesis of osteoarthritis. In: Post T, editor. UpToDate. Waltham (MA): UpToDate; 2018. Available at: www.uptodate.com. Accessed January 10, 2020.

19. Osteoarthritis Research Society International. Standardization of osteoarthritis definitions. 2015. Available at: https://www.oarsi.org/research/standardization-osteoarthritis-definitions. Accessed January 10, 2020.

20. Buys LM, Wiedenfeld SA. Osteoarthritis. In: DiPiro JT, Talbert RL, Yee GC, et al, editors. Pharmacotherapy: a pathophysiologic approach. 10e. New York: McGraw-Hill; 2017.

21. Doherty M, Bijlsma JWJ, Arden N, et al. Oxford textbook of osteoarthritis and crystal arthropathy. 3rd edition. Oxford (United Kingdom): Oxford University Press; 2016.

22. Arthritis Foundation. Arthritis by the numbers. Atlanta (GA): Arthritis Foundation; 2019. Available at: http://blog.arthritis.org/news/2019-arthritis-by-the-numbers/. Accessed January 29, 2020.

23. Vina ER, Kwoh CK. Epidemiology of osteoarthritis: literature update. Curr Opin Rheumatol 2018;30(2):160–7.

24. Spector TD, MacGregor AJ. Risk factors for osteoarthritis: genetics. Osteoarthritis Cartilage 2004;12(Suppl A):S39–44.

25. Punzi L, Galozzi P, Luisetto R, et al. Post-traumatic arthritis: overview on pathogenic mechanisms and role of inflammation. RMD Open 2016;2(2):e000279.

26. Hunter DJ, Zhang YQ, Niu JB, et al. The association of meniscal pathologic changes with cartilage loss in symptomatic knee osteoarthritis. Arthritis Rheum 2006;54(3):795–801.

27. Padua DA, DiStefano LJ, Hewett TE, et al. National athletic trainers' association position statement: prevention of anterior cruciate ligament injury. J Athl Train 2018;53(1):5–19.

28. Garstang SV, Stitik TP. Osteoarthritis: epidemiology, risk factors, and pathophysiology. Am J Phys Med Rehabil 2006;85(11 Suppl):S2–11 [quiz S12–14].

29. Jordan JM, Luta G, Renner JB, et al. Self-reported functional status in osteoarthritis of the knee in a rural southern community: the role of sociodemographic factors, obesity, and knee pain. Arthritis Care Res 1996;9(4):273–8.

30. Johns Hopkins Arthritis Center. Role of body weight in osteoarthritis. Available at: https://www.hopkinsarthritis.org/patient-corner/disease-management/role-of-body-weight-in-osteoarthritis/. Accessed January 17, 2020.

31. Guilak F. Biomechanical factors in osteoarthritis. Best Pract Res Clin Rheumatol 2011;25(6):815–23.

32. Runhaar J, Koes BW, Clockaerts S, et al. A systematic review on changed biomechanics of lower extremities in obese individuals: a possible role in development of osteoarthritis. Obes Rev 2011;12(12):1071–82.

33. Puenpatom RA, Victor TW. Increased prevalence of metabolic syndrome in individuals with osteoarthritis: an analysis of NHANES III data. Postgrad Med 2009; 121(6):9–20.

34. Le Clanche S, Bonnefont-Rousselot D, Sari-Ali E, et al. Inter-relations between osteoarthritis and metabolic syndrome: a common link? Biochimie 2016;121: 238–52.

35. Courties A, Sellam J. Osteoarthritis and type 2 diabetes mellitus: what are the links? Diabetes Res Clin Pract 2016;122:198–206.

36. Yucesoy B, Charles LE, Baker B, et al. Occupational and genetic risk factors for osteoarthritis: a review. Work 2015;50(2):261–73.

37. Cameron KL, Driban JB, Svoboda SJ. Osteoarthritis and the tactical athlete: a systematic review. J Athl Train 2016;51(11):952–61.

38. Driban JB, Hootman JM, Sitler MR, et al. Is participation in certain sports associated with knee osteoarthritis? a systematic review. J Athl Train 2017;52(6): 497–506.

39. Sharma L, Song J, Felson DT, et al. The role of knee alignment in disease progression and functional decline in knee osteoarthritis. JAMA 2001;286(2):188–95.

40. O'Reilly SC, Jones A, Muir KR, et al. Quadriceps weakness in knee osteoarthritis: the effect on pain and disability. Ann Rheum Dis 1998;57(10):588–94.

41. Bacon KL, Segal NA, Oiestad BE, et al. Thresholds in the relationship of quadriceps strength with functional limitations in women with knee osteoarthritis. Arthritis Care Res (Hoboken) 2018;71(9):1186–93.

42. McDonough CM, Jette AM. The contribution of osteoarthritis to functional limitations and disability. Clin Geriatr Med 2010;26(3):387–99.

43. Theis KA, Murphy L, Hootman JM, et al. Social participation restriction among US adults with arthritis: a population-based study using the international classification of functioning, disability and health. Arthritis Care Res (Hoboken) 2013; 65(7):1059–69.

44. Hawker GA, Stewart L, French MR, et al. Understanding the pain experience in hip and knee osteoarthritis–an OARSI/OMERACT initiative. Osteoarthritis Cartilage 2008;16(4):415–22.

45. Allen KD, Renner JB, Devellis B, et al. Osteoarthritis and sleep: the Johnston county osteoarthritis project. J Rheumatol 2008;35(6):1102–7.

46. Hunter DJ, Felson DT. Osteoarthritis. BMJ 2006;332(7542):639–42.

47. Conaghan PG, Nelson AE. Fast facts : osteoarthritis. 3rd edition. Oxford (United Kingdom): Health Press; 2017.

48. Nelson AE, Elstad E, DeVellis RF, et al. Composite measures of multi-joint symptoms, but not of radiographic osteoarthritis, are associated with functional outcomes: the Johnston county osteoarthritis project. Disabil Rehabil 2014;36(4): 300–6.

49. Block JA. Chapter 181: clinical features of osteoarthritis. In: Hochberg MC, Gravellese EM, Silman AJ, et al, editors. Rheumatology. 7th edition. Philadelphia: Elsevier; 2019. p. 1522–8.

50. Bannuru RR, Osani MC, Vaysbrot EE, et al. OARSI guidelines for the non-surgical management of knee, hip, and polyarticular osteoarthritis. Osteoarthritis Cartilage 2019;27(11):1578–89.

51. Raveendran R, Nelson AE. Lower extremity osteoarthritis: management and challenges. N C Med J 2017;78(5):332–6.

52. Hawker GA, Gignac MA, Badley E, et al. A longitudinal study to explain the pain-depression link in older adults with osteoarthritis. Arthritis Care Res (Hoboken) 2011;63(10):1382–90.

53. Axford J, Heron C, Ross F, et al. Management of knee osteoarthritis in primary care: pain and depression are the major obstacles. J Psychosom Res 2008; 64(5):461–7.

54. American Medical Society for Sports Medicine. What is a sports medicine physician? SportsMedTodaycom. 2019. Available at: https://www.sportsmedtoday.com/what-is-a-sports-medicine-physician.htm. Accessed May 23, 2019.

55. Brown GA. AAOS clinical practice guideline: treatment of osteoarthritis of the knee: evidence-based guideline, 2nd edition. J Am Acad Orthop Surg 2013; 21(9):577–9.

56. Hawker GA, Badley EM, Borkhoff CM, et al. Which patients are most likely to benefit from total joint arthroplasty? Arthritis Rheum 2013;65(5):1243–52.

57. U.S. Department of Health and Human Services. Physical activity guidelines for Americans. 2nd edition. Washington, DC: U.S. Department of Health and Human Services; 2018. Available at: https://health.gov/paguidelines/second-edition/pdf/Physical_Activity_Guidelines_2nd_edition.pdf. Accessed January 17, 2020.

58. Dunlop DD, Song J, Lee J, et al. Physical activity minimum threshold predicting improved function in adults with lower-extremity symptoms. Arthritis Care Res (Hoboken) 2017;69(4):475–83.

59. Human kinetics. Active living every day. Available at: https://us.humankinetics.com/blogs/active-living. Accessed January 16, 2020.

60. Fit & strong!. Available at: https://www.fitandstrong.org/. Accessed January 16, 2020.

61. Arthritis Foundation. Walk with ease. Available at: https://www.arthritis.org/living-with-arthritis/tools-resources/walk-with-ease/. Accessed January 16, 2020.

62. Enhance Fitness. What is EnhanceFitness?. Available at: https://projectenhance.org/enhancewellness/. Accessed January 16, 2020.

63. Messier SP, Mihalko SL, Legault C, et al. Effects of intensive diet and exercise on knee joint loads, inflammation, and clinical outcomes among overweight and obese adults with knee osteoarthritis: the IDEA randomized clinical trial. JAMA 2013;310(12):1263–73.

64. Murphy LB, Brady TJ, Boring MA, et al. Self-management education participation among US adults with arthritis: who's attending? Arthritis Care Res (Hoboken) 2017;69(9):1322–30.

65. Self-management resource center. Available at: https://www.selfmanagement resource.com/. Accessed January 16, 2020.

66. Guh DP, Zhang W, Bansback N, et al. The incidence of co-morbidities related to obesity and overweight: a systematic review and meta-analysis. BMC Public Health 2009;9:88.

67. Guglielmo D, Hootman JM, Murphy LB, et al. Health care provider counseling for weight loss among adults with arthritis and overweight or obesity - United States, 2002-2014. MMWR Morb Mortal Wkly Rep 2018;67(17):485–90.

68. Chen JC, Linnan L, Callahan LF, et al. Workplace policies and prevalence of knee osteoarthritis: the Johnston County osteoarthritis project. Occup Environ Med 2007;64(12):798–805.

69. Osteoarthritis Action Alliance. Remain in the game: a joint effort. Available at: remaininthegame.org. Accessed January 30, 2020.

70. Driban JB, Lo GH, Eaton CB, et al. Knee pain and a prior injury are associated with increased risk of a new knee injury: data from the osteoarthritis initiative. J Rheumatol 2015;42(8):1463–9.

71. Kucera KL, Marshall SW, Wolf SH, et al. Association of injury history and incident injury in cadet basic military training. Med Sci Sports Exerc 2016;48(6):1053–61.

72. Hruby A, Bulathsinhala L, McKinnon CJ, et al. BMI and lower extremity injury in US Army soldiers, 2001-2011. Am J Prev Med 2016;50(6):e163–71.

73. Kouvonen A, Kivimaki M, Oksanen T, et al. Obesity and occupational injury: a prospective cohort study of 69,515 public sector employees. PLoS One 2013;8(10): e77178.

74. National Council on Aging. Osteoarthritis and falls. Available at: https://www.ncoa.org/wp-content/uploads/osteoarthritis.-and-falls-prevention-booklet-ncoa-1.pdf. Accessed January 16, 2020.

Clinical Features, Diagnosis, and Treatment of Rheumatoid Arthritis

Ariadne V. Ebel, DO[a], James R. O'Dell, MD, MACP, MACR[b],*

KEYWORDS

- Rheumatoid arthritis • Rheumatoid factor • Anticitrullinated protein antibody
- Disease-modifying antirheumatic drug (DMARD)

KEY POINTS

- Rheumatoid arthritis (RA) is a chronic systemic autoimmune disease that is characterized by symmetric inflammatory polyarthritis and systemic inflammation.
- RA usually presents with synovitis of the small joints of the hand and feet, morning stiffness lasting more than 1 hour, and positive rheumatoid factor and/or anticitrullinated protein antibody.
- Untreated disease leads to joint deformities, significant disability, and premature death typically from cardiovascular disease.
- Early diagnosis and initiation of disease-modifying antirheumatic drug (DMARD) therapy is key to prevention of joint destruction and to decrease systemic inflammation.

INTRODUCTION AND EPIDEMIOLOGY

Rheumatoid arthritis (RA) is a chronic systemic autoimmune disease of unknown cause that primarily targets the synovial tissues. RA is characterized by symmetric inflammatory polyarthritis with systemic and extraarticular manifestations. While RA is commonly thought of as a joint disease, it is critical to realize that systemic inflammation leads to premature cardiovascular mortality. If left untreated, RA can lead to erosions, joint destruction, permanent deformities, and death. The diagnosis of RA carries a significant personal and socioeconomic burden with reduced quality of life and functional disability. Early diagnosis and treatment are key to prevention of long-term damage, morbidity, and mortality.

RA affects 0.5% to 1% of adults in developed countries. The highest rates of RA are seen in Native Americans, specifically the Pima Indians and Chippewa Indians,

[a] UCHealth Greeley Hospital, 6767 W 29th St, Greeley, CO 80634, USA; [b] Division of Rheumatology and Immunology, University of Nebraska Medical Center, Omaha Veterans Affairs, 986270 Nebraska Medical Center, Omaha, NE 68198-6270, USA
* Corresponding author.
E-mail address: jrodell@unmc.edu

Physician Assist Clin 6 (2021) 41–60
https://doi.org/10.1016/j.cpha.2020.08.004
2405-7991/21/© 2020 Elsevier Inc. All rights reserved.

physicianassistant.theclinics.com

while the lowest rates have been reported in rural African and Southeast Asia populations.[1] A study on the global burden of RA found the global prevalence rate to be 0.25% with stable prevalence rates from 1990 to 2010.[2] The cumulative lifetime risk of RA has been reported to be slightly higher for women with risk of 3.6% compared with 1.7% for men with highest incidence risk for both sexes around age 60.[3]

ETIOLOGY AND PATHOGENESIS

The pathogenesis of RA involves a complex interaction between genetic and environmental factors but the exact mechanism leading to clinical disease remains unknown. The strongest genetic risk factor for RA is the human leukocyte antigen (HLA)-DRB1 allele, which encodes major histocompatibility complex (MHC) molecules. Alleles that share a common amino acid sequence in the peptide-binding groove, referred to as the shared epitope (eg, DRB1 0401 or 0404), are strongly associated with autoreactive immune responses in RA.[4]

Smoking is a well-established risk factor for RA, especially for those with the shared epitope. Presence of the shared epitope and smoking has been shown to synergistically increase the risk of RA by 20-fold compared with nonsmokers without the shared epitope.[5] Smoking also increases RA disease activity.[6] Other environmental exposures, including silicosis and periodontitis, have been suggested to increase the risk of RA.[7,8]

Increasing evidence suggests that extraarticular mucosal sites, predominantly oral, intestinal, and lung, are the initial sites of inflammation and loss of tolerance leading to autoimmunity in RA.[9] Environmental stressors and exposures can cause injury at mucosal sites and induce peptidyl arginine deiminase, which promotes posttranslational modification of arginine to citrulline in proteins, a process referred to as citrullination. Cigarette smoke is a well-established exposure that induces citrullination in the lungs. Citrullination can also be induced by *Porphyromonas gingivalis* in periodontal disease. These citrullinated peptides bind to the shared epitope within MHC proteins with higher avidity than unmodified peptides and activate CD4 T cells more efficiently. B cells are then stimulated to produce autoantibodies, including rheumatoid factor (RF) and anticitrullinated protein antibodies (ACPAs), which recognize self-proteins and are pathogenic in RA.[10]

RF and ACPAs are found in the serum years before the onset of articular symptoms of RA. This period of autoimmunity without signs or symptoms of RA is termed "preclinical RA." The presence of autoantibodies alone is not sufficient to cause disease, although the exact mechanism that causes antibodies that have been in the serum for years to target joints remains to be elucidated. Additional immunologic events such as increasing concentrations of autoantibodies, epitope spreading, and increasing serum cytokine concentrations eventually reach a threshold that leads to synovial inflammation. Activation of various cytokines, infiltration of both innate and adaptive inflammatory cells into the synovium, immune complex formation, complement activation, and/or direct binding of autoantibodies within the synovial tissues have been proposed to contribute to RA.[11]

Synovitis results from proliferation of the synovial lining with expansion of fibroblast-like synoviocytes, which secrete proinflammatory cytokines including IL-1, IL-6, tumor necrosis factor-α (TNF-α), and matrix metalloproteinases. Synovial hyperplasia and release of these cytokines and matrix metalloproteinases leads to bone and cartilage destruction. Bone erosions also result from the activation of osteoclasts by receptor activator of nuclear factor κB ligand, IL-1, IL-6, and TNF-α.[12]

DIAGNOSIS

The diagnosis of RA is made by the combination of clinical symptoms, physical examination findings, laboratory data, and imaging. RA classically presents with pain and swelling of the small joints in the hands and feet with prolonged morning stiffness. Patients often report difficulty with activities of daily living and may experience a "gelling" phenomenon with increased stiffness after periods of rest followed by improvement in their symptoms with activity. Synovitis, tenderness, and limited range of motion may be present on joint examination.

Laboratories can be helpful for differentiating RA from other diseases and often show:

- Normal white blood cell count
- Mild normocytic anemia and thrombocytosis
- Increased erythrocyte sedimentation rate (ESR) and C-reactive protein (CRP)
- Positive RF and anticyclic citrullinated protein (anti-CCP) antibody
- Normal renal and liver function
- Normal urinalysis
- Negative antinuclear antibody (up to one-third may be positive)

RF and ACPAs (measured by using anti-CCP antibody assays) are characteristic antibodies seen in RA. RF, an autoantibody directed against the Fc portion of immunoglobulin, is positive in about 70% of patients initially and an additional 15% of patients may "seroconvert" RF^- to RF^+ later in the disease course. RF has a specificity of less than 50% and sensitivity of 70% to 80%.

ACPAs are positive in around 70% of patients but have a much higher specificity (>95%) than RF and importantly will be positive when the patients present with their symptoms. Therefore, the presence of a positive CCP antibody in a patient with an inflammatory arthritis essentially makes the diagnosis. Some individuals are negative for both RF and ACPA, which is termed "seronegative RA." Seropositivity is associated with more aggressive disease and extraarticular manifestations.

If arthrocentesis is performed, it typically shows inflammatory synovial fluid with white blood cell count ranging from 5000 to 25,000 with 60% to 80% polymorphonuclear leukocytes. Synovial culture and crystal analysis will be negative. There are no findings diagnostic for RA in the synovial fluid.

Radiographs are often normal early in the disease. Periarticular osteopenia, marginal erosions, and joint destruction can be seen on radiographs later in disease (**Figs. 1** and **2**). The characteristic erosions seen in RA are located in the "bare area" where the bone is not covered by hyaline cartilage and is exposed to the inflammatory synovium (**Fig. 3**). MRI and ultrasound have better sensitivity over conventional radiographs for detecting synovitis and erosions in early RA but are not necessary in most cases.

Technically, there are no diagnostic criteria for RA, but classification criteria are available to identify patients for clinical trials and are routinely used for diagnosis. The 1987 American College of Rheumatology (ACR) criteria and 2010 ACR/European League against Rheumatism (EULAR) criteria are shown in **Table 1**.[13] Key differences between the 1987 and 2010 criteria are that the newer criteria included laboratory data such as RF, ACPA, ESR, and CRP in addition to not requiring ≥6 weeks of joint symptoms. The new criteria produce a score from 0 to 10 with a score of ≥6 classified as definite RA. These criteria have increased the sensitivity to 97% to detect RA earlier in the disease process but have lower specificity compared with the 1987 criteria (55% versus 76%).[14]

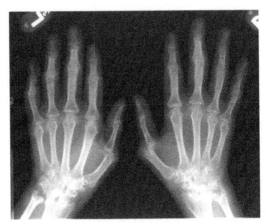

Fig. 1. Hand radiographs showing osteopenia, joint space narrowing, and progressive erosive changes typical of RA.

The differential diagnosis of RA includes many diseases that can present similarly to RA such as other connective tissue diseases, infections, and crystalline arthropathy (**Table 2**). Osteoarthritis should also be considered in the differential diagnosis and can be differentiated by symptoms, distribution of joint involvement, and laboratory and radiographic findings. Osteoarthritis is associated with joint pain that typically worsens throughout the day with increased use and involves the distal interphalangeal joints, proximal interphalangeal (PIP) joints, knees, hips, and lumbar and cervical spine (**Fig. 4**). Physical examination shows bony osteophytes with minimal soft tissue swelling and laboratories are normal. Subchondral sclerosis, osteophytes, and asymmetric joint space loss are seen on radiographs in osteoarthritis.

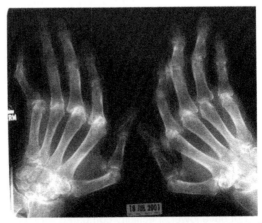

Fig. 2. Hand radiographs showing marked erosive changes and joint deformities in long-standing, suboptimally treated RA.

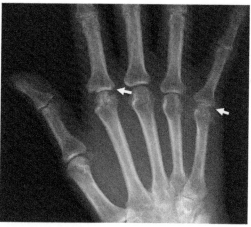

Fig. 3. Typical rheumatoid arthritis erosions (*arrows*) in RA along the "bare area."

Table 1
1987 American College of Rheumatology criteria and 2010 ACR/European League against Rheumatism criteria for classification of rheumatoid arthritis

1987 Classification Criteria: RA Present with ≥4 Criteria Present	2010 Classification Criteria: RA Present if Score ≥6 (Points)
[a]Morning stiffness >1 h	Joint involvement (includes any swollen or tender joint)[a]
[a]Arthritis of 3 joint areas	1 Urge joint (0)
[a]Arthritis of the hands	2–10 large joints (1)
[a]Symmetric arthritis	1–3 small joints (2)
Rheumatoid nodules	4–10 small joints (3)
Serum RF	>10 joints (at least 1 small joint) (5)
Typical radiographic changes	Serology[b]
[a]These criteria must be present for >6 wk	Negative RF and negative anti-CCP (0)
	Low positive RF or low positive anti-CCP (2)
	High positive RF or high positive anti-CCP (3)
	Acute phase reactants
	Normal CRP and normal ESR (0)
	Abnormal CRP or abnormal CRP (1)
	Duration of symptoms
	<6 wk (0)
	≥6 wk (1)

Abbreviations: anti-CCP, anticitrullinated peptide antibody; CRP, C-reactive protein; ESR, erythrocyte sedimentation rate; IP, interphalangeal; MCP, metacarpophalangeal; MTP, metatarsophalangeal; PIP, proximal interphalangeal; RF, rheumatoid factor; ULN, upper limit normal.
  [a] Large joints = shoulders, elbows, hips, knees and ankles; small joints = MCP, PIP, 2nd to 5th MTPs. thumb IR, and wrists.
  [b] Low positive: >ULN but < × 3 ULN; high positive > × 3 times ULN.
  Data from Arnett FC, Edworthy SM, Bloch DA, et al. The American Rheumatism Association 1987 revised criteria for the classification of rheumatoid arthritis. Arthritis Rheum. 1988;31(3):315-324. https://doi.org/10.1002/art.1780310302 and Aletaha, D., et al., 2010 Rheumatoid arthritis classification criteria: an American College of Rheumatology/European League Against Rheumatism collaborative initiative. Arthritis Rheum, 2010. 62(9): p. 2569-81.

Table 2
Rheumatoid arthritis differential diagnosis and differentiating disease features

Disease	Distinguishing Features
Other connective tissue/idiopathic forms of arthritis	
Adult-onset Still disease	Temperature >39°C for longer than 1 wk, leukocytosis >10,000/mm³ with >80% polymorphonuclear leukocytes, evanescent rash, arthralgias, sore throat, lymphadenopathy, splenomegaly, liver dysfunction, marked elevations in serum ferritin
Systemic lupus erythematosus	Nonerosive arthritis with similar joint distribution and reducible deformities (Jaccoud arthropathy), positive ANA with positive anti-dsDNA, and other serologies, ACPA⁻, associated internal organ involvement, especially the kidney
Spondyloarthropathy	Male predominance, often oligoarticular with predominantly large joint and lower extremity distribution, low back involvement, HLA-B27⁺, RF/ACPA⁻, uveitis, other associations, including psoriasis and inflammatory bowel disease
Vasculitis	Seronegative polyarthritis in a patient with systemic symptoms, such as fever, evidence of end-organ involvement; marked elevations in ESR or CRP; presence of antineutrophil cytoplasmic antibodies
Relapsing seronegative symmetric synovitis with pitting edema (RS3PE)	Marked by synovial thickening and joint tenderness with associated pitting edema of the hands, occurs in elderly men, very responsive to glucocorticoids, malignancy association; RF/ACPA⁻
Polymyalgia rheumatica	Arm and hip girdle involvement; marked elevations in ESR/CRP; RF/ACPA⁻; association with giant cell arteritis
Sarcoidosis	Acute form associated with erythema nodosum and hilar adenopathy (Lofgren syndrome), large joint involvement with a predilection for the ankle, often RF⁺ and ACPA⁻, nonerosive, pathology shows noncaseating granulomas
Sjögren syndrome	Keratoconjunctivitis sicca (dry eyes) or xerostomia (dry mouth); salivary gland enlargement; positive ANA (SS-A/SS-B), often RF⁺, ACPA⁻

(continued on next page)

Table 2 (continued)	
Disease	**Distinguishing Features**
Fibromyalgia	Myalgia without an inflammatory arthritis, RF and ACPA⁻; ESR, CRP normal
Infectious related	
Bacterial endocarditis	High fever, predominantly large joints, audible murmur, positive blood cultures, evidence of peripheral emboli; can be RF⁺, ACPA⁻
Human immunodeficiency virus	Brief acute joint pain associated with initial viremia followed by an oligoarticular process, fever
Hepatitis B and C	Nonerosive arthritis similar to RA, RF⁺, ACPA⁻, hypocomplementemia, positive HBV/HCV serologies, cryoglobulins
Parvovirus B19	Nonerosive arthritis typically seronegative, self-limited process, parvovirus IgM⁺, viral presentation
Chikungunya	Insect-borne virus, acute febrile illness with rash followed by a polyarthritis
Poststreptococcal infection	Nonerosive arthritis in a patient with an antecedent skin or oropharynx group A streptococcal infection, antistreptolysin O⁺
Rheumatic fever	Polyarthritis that is often additive, symmetric, with large joint lower extremity involvement; subcutaneous nodules, carditis, chorea, rash
Lyme disease	May have both an erosive and nonerosive arthritis, RF, and ACPA⁻, history of a tick bite and/or typical rash while in an endemic region
Crystalline arthropathy	
Calcium pyrophosphate dihydrate deposition disease	Often in elderly women, 5% incidence of pseudo-RA presentation, radiographs may have chondrocalcinosis; associations with hemochromatosis, hyperparathyroidism, hypothyroidism, and hypomagnesemia
Polyarticular gout	Often involves distal joints, including first MTP, and may affect the DIP joints of the hands, associated tophaceous nodules, RF/ACPA⁻, erosions with "overhanging edge"; hyperuricemia

(continued on next page)

Table 2 (continued)	
Disease	**Distinguishing Features**
Systemic manifestations of other medical conditions	
Thyroid disease	Polyarthralgias and myalgias with other manifestations of thyroid disease; carpal tunnel symptoms may be present
Malignancy	Often represents a paraneoplastic process and can mimic RA; lymphoma can present like RA; may be RF+ but usually ACPA−
Hypertrophic osteoarthropathy	Predominant involvement in knees, ankles, wrists; associations with chronic lung disease (eg, cystic fibrosis) and malignancy; bone pain and periostitis

Abbreviations: ACPA, anticitrullinated protein antibodies; ANA, antinuclear antibody; CRP, C-reactive protein; ESR, erythrocyte sedimentation rate; DIP, distal interphalangeal; HLA, human leukocyte antigen; MTP, metatarsophalangeal.

From O'Dell, J. et al, *Clinical features of rheumatoid arthritis,* in *Kelley & Firestein's Textbook of Rheumatology,* G.S. Firestein, Budd R. C., Gabriel S. E., McInnes I.B., O'Dell J.R., Editor. 2017, Elsevier Saunders: Philadelphia. p. 1170; with permission.

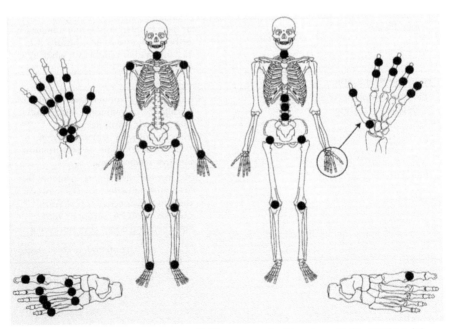

Fig. 4. Typical joint distributions in RA (*left*) compared with osteoarthritis (OA) (*right*).

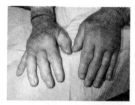

Fig. 5. Symmetric synovitis in the metacarpophalangeal (MCP) and proximal interphalangeal (PIP) joints.

CLINICAL MANIFESTATIONS
Articular Manifestations

The classic distribution of RA involves the small joints of the hands and feet and this is reflected in the new classification criteria (see **Table 1**). The metacarpophalangeal (MCP), PIP, and metatarsophalangeal (MTP) joints are typically involved with associated morning stiffness, joint pain, and swelling (see **Fig. 4; Fig. 5**). Morning stiffness is a classic sign of inflammatory arthritis and often lasts more than an hour. Other synovial joints may be involved over time, especially if therapy is delayed, and include the wrists, knees, elbows, ankles, hips, shoulders, and cervical spine (C1-C2). Appropriate treatment can prevent the spread of RA to proximal joints. The distal interphalangeal (DIP) joints and thoracic and lumbosacral spine are spared in RA.

RA onset varies from acute to insidious. Insidious onset of symmetric arthritis of the small joints of the wrist, hands, and feet is the most common. RA can also present similarly to a seronegative spondyloarthropathy with insidious onset of monoarticular or oligoarticular arthritis with additional small joint and symmetric involvement over time. Less frequently, RA can present acutely with an intense inflammatory polyarticular arthritis in which patients may seek urgent attention. Palindromic rheumatism is another pattern of onset characterized by brief, self-limited episodes of severe joint inflammation most commonly affecting the shoulders, knees, and fingers. Up to half of palindromic patients will eventually evolve to a pattern more characteristic of RA. Rarely, RA can present with extraarticular manifestations at disease onset such as interstitial lung disease (ILD).

Progressive inflammation and damage to the joints and surrounding tendons results in the classic "zigzag" deformity with ulnar deviation and palmar subluxation of the MCP joints and radial deviation of the wrist (**Fig. 6**). Other well-recognized deformities, swan neck and boutonnière deformities, result from stretching of ligaments and tendons (**Figs. 7 and 8**). Swan neck deformities result from DIP flexion and PIP

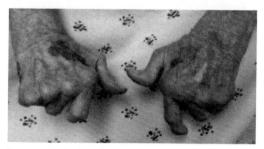

Fig. 6. "Zigzag" deformity of the hand with radial deviation at the wrist and subluxation and ulnar deviation at the MCP joints.

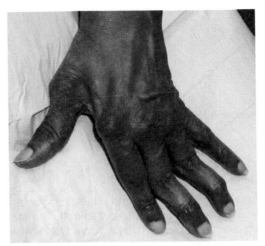

Fig. 7. Swan neck deformity: hyperextension of the proximal interphalangeal joint and flexion of the distal interphalangeal joints.

hyperextension and boutonnière deformities from PIP flexion and DIP hyperextension. Tenosynovitis in the flexor tendon sheaths in the hands can cause hand weakness or median nerve impingement resulting in carpal tunnel syndrome. Thickening of the tendon sheaths can lead to "trigger finger," which causes the finger to lock in flexion. Rupture of the extensor tendons of the hands can occur most typically at the ulnar head in the wrist. The extensor digiti minimi usually ruptures first and can be tested for by independent extension of the fifth digit. Fortunately, these complications are now rarely seen with earlier diagnosis and initiation of disease-modifying antirheumatic drug (DMARD) therapy.

Synovitis of the MTP joints is common in RA and patients often describe the symptoms as "walking on marbles." Claw toe deformities of the PIP joints may result from

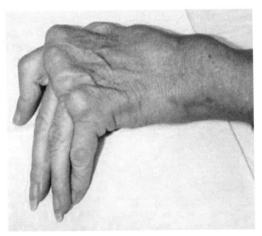

Fig. 8. MCP subluxation and boutonnière deformity of the second digit: flexion of the proximal interphalangeal joint and extension of the distal interphalangeal joint.

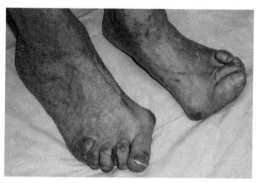

Fig. 9. Pes planus, severe hallux valgus, claw toe, and cross-over deformities of the toes.

plantar subluxation of the metatarsal heads leading to callus formation. The ankle, hindfoot, and midfoot are also commonly involved and can lead to valgus and pes planus deformities (**Fig. 9**).

The top of the cervical spine is also often involved in RA and is most commonly seen in patients with long-standing disease. Atlantoaxial (C1-C2) subluxation is the most serious manifestation because of potential spinal cord compression (**Fig. 10**). Any

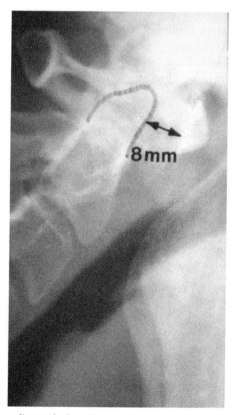

Fig. 10. Cervical spine radiograph showing anterior subluxation of C1 on C2.

RA patients, particularly those with hand deformities, planning to undergo surgery or anesthesia should have flexion and extension radiographs to screen for C1-C2 subluxation because fatal subluxation may result from forced flexion of the cervical spine.

Extraarticular Manifestations

Extraarticular manifestations typically occur with more long-standing disease but rarely can be the initial presentation of RA. Systemic manifestations, particularly fatigue, low-grade fever, and weight loss, may be present in early disease. Patients with extraarticular manifestations tend to be seropositive and have higher morbidity and mortality. Some of the more common extraarticular manifestations are listed below:

- Mucocutaneous:
  - Rheumatoid nodules—subcutaneous nodules most common on extensor surfaces in seropositive patients (**Fig. 11**)
  - Secondary Sjögren syndrome
  - Vasculitis, very rarely amyloidosis or pyoderma gangrenosum
- Ocular:
  - Secondary Sjögren syndrome
  - Episcleritis and scleritis
- Cardiovascular disease
  - Atherosclerosis (myocardial infarction, congestive heart failure, stroke)
  - Pericarditis and pericardial effusions
- Pulmonary:
  - ILD (usual interstitial pneumonia [UIP] pattern most common)
  - Obstructive lung disease
  - Rheumatoid nodules
  - Exudative pleural effusion (usually asymptomatic)
- Hematologic:
  - Normocytic anemia and thrombocytosis
  - Felty syndrome (triad of RA, splenomegaly, and leukopenia)
  - Large granular lymphocyte syndrome (profound neutropenia)
- Vasculitis:
  - Rheumatoid nodules
  - Small to medium vessel vasculitis (skin and peripheral nervous system most frequently involved with life-threatening PAN picture)

Complications

Some of the more severe extraarticular manifestations of RA, including ILD, cardiovascular disease, and malignancy, are associated with increased mortality. Patients with RA have an increased risk of lymphoma (2-fold) and lung cancer compared with the

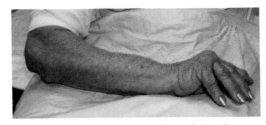

Fig. 11. Rheumatoid nodule over the extensor surface of the elbow.

general population.[15] The risk of lymphoma in RA seems to be predominately associated with increased disease activity rather than from immunosuppressive therapy.[16] Cardiovascular disease is the leading cause of mortality in RA, is correlated with disease activity, and is not completely explained by the traditional risk factors.[17] ILD is the most severe pulmonary complication in RA and most common pulmonary cause of death. UIP is the most common subtype in RA. Male sex, older age, cigarette smoking, and autoantibody positivity are risk factors for RA-associated ILD.[18]

RA patients are at higher risk of osteoporosis and fragility fractures. The vertebral spine is the most common site of fracture in RA patients. RA is considered to be an independent risk factor for osteoporosis in the fracture risk assessment tool used to calculate 10-year risk of major osteoporotic fracture and hip fracture. Duration of RA, disease activity, and steroid use are RA-specific factors that have been found to contribute to fracture risk.[19]

MANAGEMENT

There have been truly dramatic improvements in outcomes in RA over the last quarter century due to earlier recognition of disease and advancement in treatment strategies. Early diagnosis and initiation of DMARD therapy at the time of diagnosis are key to preventing joint damage and disability. The goal and expectation for most patients diagnosed currently with RA should be remission of RA on therapy. Use of optimal doses of methotrexate (MTX) with folic acid, combinations of DMARDs, biologics, and, most importantly, treating all patients to a disease activity target, are changes over the years that have contributed to improved outcomes. Currently 23 DMARDs are available to treat RA and they are often used together, resulting in a daunting number of possible combinations (>10,000). Obviously, discussion of all of these is beyond the scope of this article so please refer to the following references.[20–29]

In a treat-to-target approach for RA, disease activity is reassessed routinely and therapy is adjusted to achieve low disease activity or remission.[30,31] There is no specific laboratory test for monitoring disease activity in RA but there are various composite disease activity tools that can be used in clinical practice in a treat-to-target approach. The Clinical Disease Activity Index, Simplified Disease Activity Index, Routine Assessment Patient Index Data, and Disease Activity Score in 28 joints incorporate information from the joint examination, patient function, patient and physician assessment of disease activity, and inflammatory markers to assess disease activity. It is most important that disease activity is measured and less important which instrument is used because each disease activity instrument has strengths and limitations.

The goals of treatment of RA are to prevent joint damage and disease complications as well as improve the patient's quality of life and function. The decision on which specific therapy to use to achieve these goals is not as crucial as initiating treatment early and that the specific treatment meets the low disease activity or remission target. The choice of DMARD should be individualized for each patient, taking into account disease activity, comorbidities, cost, and patient preferences. At this time there are no parameters or biomarkers that predict which patients will have optimal responses to each medication so there is no one right answer for which DMARD to use.[23] The approach to treatment of RA recommended by the American College of Rheumatology is included in **Fig. 12**.[32]

DMARDs have been shown to improve the clinical course and radiographic progression of RA and are divided into conventional synthetic and biologic therapies. Biosimilar DMARDs are considered equivalent in effectiveness and safety to the original biologics. MTX, sulfasalazine, hydroxychloroquine, and leflunomide are the

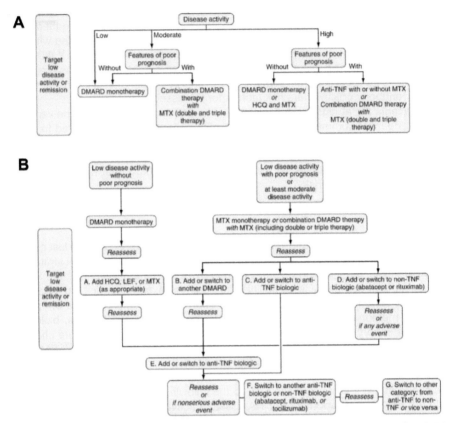

Fig. 12. American College of Rheumatology recommendations for rheumatoid arthritis treatment in early disease (*A*) and established disease (*B*). (*From* O'Dell, J. et al, Treatment of rheumatoid arthritis. In: Firestein GS, Budd RC, Gabriel SE, et al, eds. Kelley & Firestein's Textbook of Rheumatology, 2017, Elsevier: Philadelphia. p, 1195; with permission.)

most commonly used conventional DMARDs and are often used in combination with other conventional or biologic DMARDs. Biologic DMARDs inhibit specific inflammatory cytokines including TNF, IL-6, and IL-1, as well as B and T cells. Refer to **Tables 3** and **4** for more information on each specific DMARD.

MTX is the initial therapy of choice for RA and is the foundation for managing RA for most patients.[27,33,34] MTX is inexpensive and can be effective as monotherapy. Most DMARDs are more effective when combined with MTX, especially anti-TNF therapy.[35,36] The optimal doses of MTX for RA (up to 25 mg once weekly) are generally well tolerated if administered along with daily folic acid.[37] Importantly, in the rheumatology world, MTX is always a 1 day a week therapy. Patients should be monitored for toxicity including bone marrow suppression, hepatotoxicity, and the rare pneumonitis. MTX is cleared by the kidney so patients with chronic kidney disease 4 or 5 are not MTX candidates, and creatinine should be followed while a patient is on MTX. MTX is teratogenic so it should not be prescribed to those planning to conceive in the near future. MTX can be administered orally but the subcutaneous route is more effective due to better bioavailability. More than 50% of patients will achieve low disease activity or remission with subcutaneous MTX monotherapy.[38]

Table 3
Synthetic disease-modifying antirheumatic drugs for rheumatoid arthritis

Drug	Dose/Route	Mechanism of Action	Side Effects
Methotrexate	7.5–25 mg/wk po/SQ	Inhibits dihydrofolate reductase, increase release of adenosine that inhibits inflammation	Stomatitis Nausea/vomiting Increased LFTs Cytopenia Pneumonitis contraindicated in pregnancy and CrCl < 30
Sulfasalazine	1–3 g/d po	Anti-inflammatory and immunomodulatory properties. Metabolized to sulfapyradine and 5-ASA	Rash Nausea/vomiting Diarrhea Neutropenia Reversible azoospermia
Hydroxychloroquine	200–400 mg/d (<5 mg/kg)	Anti-inflammatory and immunomodulatory properties.	Retinal toxicity (late) Myopathy/ neuropathy Hypoglycemia
Leflunomide	10–20 mg/d	Inhibits dihydroorotate dehydrogenase	Nausea/vomiting Diarrhea Rash Cytopenia Hepatic toxicity Contraindicated in pregnancy
Doxycycline Minocycline	100 mg bid 100 mg bid	Inhibit metalloproteinase and modulate immune responses	Lightheadedness Drug-induced lupus and cutaneous hyperpigmenta-tion (minocycline)
Tofacitinib Baricitinib Upadacitinib	5 mg po bid 2 mg po qd 15 mg po qd	JAK inhibitor	Infection Herpes zoster Cytopenia Increased LFTs Thrombosis Gastrointestinal perforation

Abbreviation: LFT, liver function test.

Combinations of DMARDs are often needed to adequately control disease.[39–41] If a patient continues to have active disease despite MTX then another DMARD should be added to MTX rather than discontinuing it. The strategy of adding sulfasalazine and hydroxychloroquine to MTX (triple therapy) has been shown to be noninferior to adding etanercept (TNF inhibitor),[42] supporting the approach of starting biologic therapy after combinations of conventional DMARDs fail. Patients who are refractory to conventional DMARDs and TNF inhibitors have many other options with different mechanisms of action including B-cell depletion (rituximab), T-cell modulation (abatacept), IL-6 inhibition (tocilizumab and sarilumab), or Jak inhibition (tofacitinib, baricitinib, and

Table 4
Biological disease-modifying antirheumatic drugs for rheumatoid arthritis

Drug	Dose/Route	Mechanism of Action	Side Effects

Adalimumab
Certolizumab
Etanercept
Golimumab
 	
Infliximab
	40 mg SQ Q2 week
	200 mg SQ Q2 week
	50 mg SQ weekly
	50 mg SQ monthly or
	  2 mg/kg IV Q8 week
	3 mg/kg to 10 mg/kg
	  Q 4 to Q 8
		TNF inhibitor	Injection site reaction
			Infusion reactions (IV)
			Infection (screen for TB and
			  hepatitis B)
			Congestive heart failure
			  exacerbation
			Drug-induced lupus
			Contraindicated in demyelinating
			  disease and malignancy

Tocilizumab
Sarilumab
	<100 kg: 162 mg SQ QOW,
	  can increase to weekly
	≥100 kg: 162 mg SQ Qweek
	4 mg/kg IV Q4 week
	200 mg SQ Q2 week
		IL-6 receptor
		  antagonist
			Infections
			Injection site reaction
			Infusion reactions
			Increased LFTs
			Neutropenia
			Thrombocytopenia
			Lipid elevation
			Gastrointestinal perforation

Abatacept	125 mg SQ weekly
	<60 kg: 500 mg IV
	60–100 kg: 750 mg IV
	>100 kg: 1000 mg IV
	Q4 weeks
		T-cell co-
		  stimulation
		  modulator
			Infections
			Chronic obstructive
			  pulmonary disease
			  exacerbation
			Injection site reaction
			Infusion reaction

Rituximab	1000 mg IV ×2 doses
	  (14 d apart)
		Anti-CD20
		  monoclonal
		  antibody
			Infusion reaction
			Infection
			Hypogammaglobulinemia
			Neutropenia
			PML

Anakinra	100 mg SQ daily	IL-1 receptor antagonist	Injection site reaction Infection Neutropenia

Abbreviation: LFT, liver function test.

upadacitinib).[24–27] Biologic agents and Jaks should not be combined due to increased risk of infections.

Nonsteroidal anti-inflammatory drugs (NSAIDs) may reduce symptoms of pain and stiffness by inhibiting prostaglandin synthesis but do not prevent joint damage; therefore, NSAIDs should not be used as monotherapy in RA without DMARDs. Glucocorticoids are potent and rapid-acting DMARDs but, due to universal long-term side effects, should be used at the lowest dose and shortest time possible.[28] Glucocorticoids should only be used with other DMARDs and as a short-term bridge to allow the other DMARD time to work. Side effects of long-term glucocorticoids include osteoporosis, infection, hypertension, hyperglycemia, glaucoma, and cataracts, are dose dependent but over time occur in essentially all patients.

THE ROLE OF PRIMARY CARE PROVIDERS

Optimal care of RA patients requires a team-based approach between primary care providers, including physicians and advanced practice providers, and rheumatologists.

DMARDs and biologics require regular monitoring by the rheumatologist with frequent laboratories to screen bone marrow and liver toxicity, as well as annual eye examinations to screen for retinal toxicity if on hydroxychloroquine. However, the primary care provider will often see RA patients first for complications or toxicity such as infection and MTX pneumonitis, so it is important that these complications are recognized and DMARD therapy is withheld while further workup is completed.

Nonpharmacologic therapies are also important in the management of RA.[29] Smoking cessation and treatment of hypertension, hyperlipidemia, and diabetes should be addressed by primary care providers to reduce the risk of cardiovascular disease. Smoking is also associated with increased disease activity and decreased efficacy of DMARD therapy. Immunizations, including annual influenza, pneumococcal, and varicella zoster vaccines, are recommended to decrease risk of infection while on immunosuppressive therapies. These immunizations can be safely administered to patients on biologic agents but ideally should be administered before starting DMARD therapy for optimal immunologic response. Live vaccinations should be given with caution in patients on biologics. Patients should also be screened and treated for osteoporosis, especially patients taking glucocorticoids.

Guidelines for DMARD management in the perioperative periods recommend that conventional synthetic DMARDs are continued throughout the perioperative period in patients undergoing elective total hip arthroplasty (THA) or total knee arthroplasty (TKA). Biologic DMARDs should be withheld 1 dosing cycle before elective THA or TKA and restarted once wound healing is achieved.[43] These recommendations on management of DMARDs in the perioperative period are often extrapolated to other elective surgical procedures.

OUTCOMES AND UNMET NEEDS

The prognosis for RA patients has improved dramatically because RA is diagnosed and treated earlier with a treat-to-target approach. The need for joint surgeries and extraarticular complications has decreased over the years as a result of more aggressive treatment targets. Most patients who take DMARDs can be expected to achieve low disease activity or remission; however, some patients may not reach these goals and further advancements in the therapies are needed. One of the biggest challenges is having parameters that predict for each individual patient which medication or combination would be best. Therefore, further research is needed to identify specific biomarkers or individual patient parameters that could be used to help personalize therapy. Fortunately, many patients do obtain remission, so the question of how and when to titrate DMARDs in these patients is now an important one. Unfortunately, patient compliance and access to medications remains a significant issue without easy answers.

SUMMARY

RA is a systemic autoimmune disease characterized by inflammatory arthritis and extraarticular manifestations including premature cardiovascular deaths. The diagnosis should be made early and treatment with DMARDs should be initiated expeditiously. Early diagnosis and the advancement in therapeutic options have contributed to dramatically improved outcomes in RA. While unanswered questions, particularly in optimizing therapy for each patient remain, patients treated early by an effective team consisting of a rheumatologist and a primary care physician or advanced practice provider have an excellent prognosis.

CLINICS CARE POINTS

- Early diagnosis is critical and swollen joint plus CCP positivity = RA.
- All RA patients should be seeing a rheumatologist.
- Methotrexate is foundation of all RA treatment and is always only once per week.
- Methotrexate is more effective and better tolerated subcutaneously.
- Biologics are wonderful but only 30 to 40% of patients should need them.

DISCLOSURE

The authors have nothing to disclose.

REFERENCES

1. Silman AJ, Pearson JE. Epidemiology and genetics of rheumatoid arthritis. Arthritis Res 2002;4(Suppl 3):S265–72.
2. Cross M, Smith E, Hoy D, et al. The global burden of rheumatoid arthritis: estimates from the global burden of disease 2010 study. Ann Rheum Dis 2014; 73(7):1316–22.
3. Crowson CS, Matteson EL, Myasoedova E, et al. The lifetime risk of adult-onset rheumatoid arthritis and other inflammatory autoimmune rheumatic diseases. Arthritis Rheum 2011;63(3):633–9.
4. Gregersen PK, Silver J, Winchester RJ. The shared epitope hypothesis. An approach to understanding the molecular genetics of susceptibility to rheumatoid arthritis. Arthritis Rheum 1987;30(11):1205–13.
5. Kallberg H, Ding B, Padyukov L, et al. Smoking is a major preventable risk factor for rheumatoid arthritis: estimations of risks after various exposures to cigarette smoke. Ann Rheum Dis 2011;70(3):508–11.
6. Sokolove J, Wagner CA, Lahey LJ, et al. Increased inflammation and disease activity among current cigarette smokers with rheumatoid arthritis: a cross-sectional analysis of US veterans. Rheumatology (Oxford) 2016;55(11):1969–77.
7. Mikuls TR, Payne JB, Yu F, et al. Periodontitis and *Porphyromonas gingivalis* in patients with rheumatoid arthritis. Arthritis Rheumatol 2014;66(5):1090–100.
8. Stolt P, Källberg H, Lundberg I, et al. Silica exposure is associated with increased risk of developing rheumatoid arthritis: results from the Swedish EIRA study. Ann Rheum Dis 2005;64(4):582–6.
9. Demoruelle MK, Deane KD, Holers VM. When and where does inflammation begin in rheumatoid arthritis? Curr Opin Rheumatol 2014;26(1):64–71.
10. Hill JA, Southwood S, Sette A, et al. Cutting edge: the conversion of arginine to citrulline allows for a high-affinity peptide interaction with the rheumatoid arthritis-associated HLA-DRB1*0401 MHC class II molecule. J Immunol 2003; 171(2):538–41.
11. Arend WP, Firestein GS. Pre-rheumatoid arthritis: predisposition and transition to clinical synovitis. Nat Rev Rheumatol 2012;8(10):573–86.
12. McInnes IB, Schett G. The pathogenesis of rheumatoid arthritis. N Engl J Med 2011;365(23):2205–19.
13. Aletaha D, Neogi T, Silman AJ, et al. 2010 Rheumatoid Arthritis Classification Criteria: an American College of Rheumatology/European League Against Rheumatism collaborative initiative. Arthritis Rheum 2010;62(9):2569–81.
14. Kennish L, Labitigan M, Budoff S, et al. Utility of the new Rheumatoid Arthritis 2010 ACR/EULAR classification criteria in routine clinical care. BMJ Open 2012;2(5):e001117.

15. Simon TA, Thompson A, Gandhi KK, et al. Incidence of malignancy in adult patients with rheumatoid arthritis: a meta-analysis. Arthritis Res Ther 2015;17:212.

16. Baecklund E, Ekbom A, Sparén P, et al. Disease activity and risk of lymphoma in patients with rheumatoid arthritis: nested case-control study. Bmj 1998; 317(7152):180–1.

17. England BR, Sayles H, Michaud K, et al. Cause-specific mortality in male US veterans with rheumatoid arthritis. Arthritis Care Res (Hoboken) 2016;68(1):36–45.

18. Kelly CA, Saravanan V, Nisar M, et al. Rheumatoid arthritis-related interstitial lung disease: associations, prognostic factors and physiological and radiological characteristics—a large multicentre UK study. Rheumatology (Oxford) 2014; 53(9):1676–82.

19. Jin S, Hsieh E, Peng L, et al. Incidence of fractures among patients with rheumatoid arthritis: a systematic review and meta-analysis. Osteoporos Int 2018;29(6): 1263–75.

20. O'Dell J. Treatment of rheumatoid arthritis. In: Firestein GS, Budd RC, Gabriel SE, et al, editors. Kelley & Firestein's textbook of rheumatology. Philadelphia: Elsevier Saunders; 2017. p. 1187–212.

21. Mcinnes I, O'Dell J. Rheumatoid arthritis. In: Goldman L, Schafer AI, editors. Goldman-Cecil medicine. Philadelphia: Elsevier; 2019. Chapter 248.

22. Moreland LW, Cannella A. General principles of management of rheumatoid arthritis. In: O'Dell JR, editor. UpToDate. Waltham (MA): 2019.

23. Cohen S, Mikuls TR. Initial treatment of rheumatoid arthritis in adults. In: O'Dell JR, editor. UpToDate. Waltham (MA): Walters Kluwer; 2019.

24. Cohen S, Cannella A. Treatment of rheumatoid arthritis in adults resistant to initial conventional nonbiologic DMARD therapy. In: O'Dell JR, editor. UpToDate. Waltham (MA): Walters Kluwer; 2019.

25. Cohen S, Mikuls TR. Alternatives to methotrexate for the initial treatment of rheumatoid arthritis in adults. In: O'Dell JR, editor. UpToDate. Waltham (MA): Walters Kluwer; 2019.

26. Cohen S, Cannella A. Treatment of rheumatoid arthritis in adults resistant to initial biologic DMARD therapy. In: O'Dell JR, editor. UpToDate. Waltham (MA): Walters Kluwer; 2019.

27. Kremer JM. Use of methotrexate in the treatment of rheumatoid arthritis. In: O'Dell JR, editor. UpToDate. Waltham (MA): Walters Kluwer; 2019.

28. O'Dell JR, Matteson EL. Use of glucocorticoids in the treatment of rheumatoid arthritis. In: St. Clair EW, editor. UpToDate. Waltham (MA): Walters Kluwer; 2019.

29. Schur PH, Gibofsky A. Nonpharmacologic therapies and preventive measures for patients with rheumatoid arthritis. In: O'Dell JR, editor. UpToDate. Waltham (MA): Walters Kluwer; 2019.

30. Grigor C, Capell H, Stirling A, et al. Effect of a treatment strategy of tight control for rheumatoid arthritis (the TICORA study): a single-blind randomised controlled trial. Lancet 2004;364(9430):263–9.

31. Mierau M, Schoels M, Gonda G, et al. Assessing remission in clinical practice. Rheumatology (Oxford) 2007;46(6):975–9.

32. Singh JA, Saag KG, Bridges SL, et al. 2015 American College of Rheumatology Guideline for the Treatment of Rheumatoid Arthritis. Arthritis Care Res (Hoboken) 2016;68(1):1–25.

33. Weinblatt ME. Efficacy of methotrexate in rheumatoid arthritis. Br J Rheumatol 1995;34(Suppl 2):43–8.

34. Visser K, van der Heijde D. Optimal dosage and route of administration of methotrexate in rheumatoid arthritis: a systematic review of the literature. Ann Rheum Dis 2009;68(7):1094–9.

35. Breedveld FC, Weisman MH, Kavanaugh AF, et al. The PREMIER study: a multicenter, randomized, double-blind clinical trial of combination therapy with adalimumab plus methotrexate versus methotrexate alone or adalimumab alone in patients with early, aggressive rheumatoid arthritis who had not had previous methotrexate treatment. Arthritis Rheum 2006;54(1):26–37.

36. van der Heijde D, Klareskog L, Rodriguez-Valverde V, et al. Comparison of etanercept and methotrexate, alone and combined, in the treatment of rheumatoid arthritis: two-year clinical and radiographic results from the TEMPO study, a double-blind, randomized trial. Arthritis Rheum 2006;54(4):1063–74.

37. van Ede AE, Laan RF, Rood MJ, et al. Effect of folic or folinic acid supplementation on the toxicity and efficacy of methotrexate in rheumatoid arthritis: a forty-eight week, multicenter, randomized, double-blind, placebo-controlled study. Arthritis Rheum 2001;44(7):1515–24.

38. O'Connor A, Thorne C, Kang H, et al. The rapid kinetics of optimal treatment with subcutaneous methotrexate in early inflammatory arthritis: an observational study. BMC Musculoskelet Disord 2016;17(1):364.

39. Elliott MJ, Maini RN, Feldmann M, et al. Randomised double-blind comparison of chimeric monoclonal antibody to tumour necrosis factor alpha (cA2) versus placebo in rheumatoid arthritis. Lancet 1994;344(8930):1105–10.

40. O'Dell JR, Haire CE, Erikson N, et al. Treatment of rheumatoid arthritis with methotrexate alone, sulfasalazine and hydroxychloroquine, or a combination of all three medications. N Engl J Med 1996;334(20):1287–91.

41. Goekoop-Ruiterman YP, de Vries-Bouwstra JK, Allaart CF, et al. Clinical and radiographic outcomes of four different treatment strategies in patients with early rheumatoid arthritis (the BeSt study): a randomized, controlled trial. Arthritis Rheum 2005;52(11):3381–90.

42. O'Dell JR, Mikuls TR, Taylor TH, et al. Therapies for active rheumatoid arthritis after methotrexate failure. N Engl J Med 2013;369(4):307–18.

43. Goodman SM, Springer B, Guyatt G, et al. 2017 American College of Rheumatology/American Association of Hip and Knee Surgeons Guideline for the perioperative management of antirheumatic medication in patients with rheumatic diseases undergoing elective total hip or total knee arthroplasty. Arthritis Care Res (Hoboken) 2017;69(8):1538–51.

Systemic Lupus Erythematosus

A Complex, but Recognizable and Treatable Disease

Benjamin J Smith, DMSc, PA-C

KEYWORDS

- Systemic lupus erythematosus • Antinuclear antibody • Autoantibodies
- Hydroxychloroquine

KEY POINTS

- SLE is a chronic, systemic, autoimmune disease that requires vigilant health care follow-up for best patient outcomes.
- A thorough history and physical examination are essential when considering SLE as a diagnosis.
- System review laboratory, such as a complete blood count (CBC), metabolic profiles including renal function laboratory, and urinalysis, are necessary for initial diagnosis and monitoring of individuals with SLE.
- Although helpful in diagnosing SLE, a positive antinuclear antibody (ANA) is only one piece of the SLE diagnostic puzzle.
- Pharmacologic and nonpharmacologic treatment options are important for persons with SLE.

INTRODUCTION

Systemic lupus erythematosus (SLE) is a chronic, inflammatory autoimmune condition that has the potential to affect multiple organ systems. SLE is described as a protean condition because it affects individuals in various and unique ways. Some patients present with mild symptoms, whereas others present with severe, life-threatening manifestations. Because of the potential to affect various body systems and with varying levels of disease activity, SLE can present as a diagnostic and treatment dilemma for health care providers. This article reviews the spectrum of disease manifestations of SLE, the diagnostic approach when SLE is suspected, and the pharmacologic and nonpharmacologic treatment options for this condition.

Florida State University College of Medicine, School of Physician Assistant Practice, 1115 West Call Street, Tallahassee, FL 32306-4300, USA
E-mail address: benjamin.smith@med.fsu.edu

Physician Assist Clin 6 (2021) 61–73
https://doi.org/10.1016/j.cpha.2020.08.005
2405-7991/21/© 2020 Elsevier Inc. All rights reserved.

LOOKING BACK IN THE MEDICAL HISTORY BOOKS

Lupus in Latin means wolf. The term lupus was used initially to describe the appearance of the notable cutaneous changes because these skin changes appeared similar to those of an animal bite.[1,2] Hippocrates described a "gnawing dermatosis" that some consider to be an early description of lupus.[3]

Over subsequent centuries as medical science advanced, so too did the understanding of the clinical manifestations of SLE. In the late 1800s, the systemic signs of SLE were recognized. The famed Sir William Osler also had a role in the history of lupus recognizing dermatologic, cardiac, pulmonary, and renal manifestations of lupus. He is noted for first using the term "systemic lupus erythematosus."[4] Many other physicians and scientists are credited with further describing SLE.

LE cells were discovered in 1948 by Dr Malcolm Hargraves, a Mayo Clinic hematologist.[5] Other laboratory science discoveries in the twentieth century helped to advance the diagnostic tools available for SLE.

IS IT SYSTEMIC LUPUS ERYTHEMATOSUS?

There are several autoimmune disorders that are defined by their clinical and serologic features. SLE is the prototypical systemic autoimmune condition, but there are other systemic autoimmune conditions, such as Sjögren syndrome, systemic sclerosis, and inflammatory myopathies, some of which are discussed elsewhere in this issue. Although some treatments for SLE and the other systemic autoimmune diseases are similar, it is important to recognize and distinguish the specific features of a person's presentation to develop a unique treatment plan for each patient.

The focus of this article is SLE. There are other recognized diagnoses that include lupus in their name. Subacute cutaneous lupus erythematosus (SCLE) is a condition that affects the skin. Usually patients with SCLE have a negative antinuclear antibody (ANA), but may have positive Sjögren antibodies (SS-A and/or SS-B). Although a person with primary SCLE may not have other features to support an SLE diagnosis, SCLE is a manifestation for persons with SLE.

Discoid lupus erythematosus is another subset condition with the word lupus in its name. Although discoid lupus has been part of the SLE classification criteria, some patients only have discoid lesions without other systemic lupus features. Discoid lesions are described as patches that are raised and erythematous with adherent keratotic scaling and follicular plugging. Chronic discoid lesions may become atrophic and scar.

SYSTEMIC LUPUS ERYTHEMATOSUS BY THE NUMBERS

Persons with SLE are found worldwide, although at differing incidence and prevalence. In North America, the incidence is reported as 23.2 per 100,000 person-years with a prevalence of 241 per 100,000 people.[6] Persons with African ethnicity have the highest incidence and prevalence. White persons have the lowest incidence and prevalence.[1] Registries from the United States show high prevalence and incidence in African Americans, American Indian, Alaska Native, Hispanic, and Asian populations.[7-11]

Women of childbearing age are more commonly affected by SLE, but men are also diagnosed with SLE. A study from Spain suggests differences among females and males with SLE. In this study, female patients with lupus tended to have more inflammatory rashes, alopecia, Raynaud phenomenon, and arthritis. Men tended to have the following features: cardiovascular comorbidities, frequent hospitalizations, weight loss, lupus nephritis, lymphadenopathy, splenomegaly, and pulmonary fibrosis. Additionally, men tend to be older at the age of diagnosis, but had a shorter diagnosis delay. This study also suggested that patients with pulmonary hemorrhage, pulmonary hypertension, psychiatric involvement, complement deficiency, and hematologic manifestations tended to have a higher mortality rate.[12]

CAUSE

The underlying cause of SLE is not known, but is believed to be multifactorial including influences from genetic predisposition, environmental contributors, and behavioral factors. Environmental and behavioral variables are discussed later in this article.

SYMPTOMS AND SIGNS

The features an individual with SLE manifests, whether subjective or objective, are often different when compared with another person with SLE. SLE symptoms and signs may occur suddenly or may develop insidiously over time. **Table 1** provides a summary of a percentage of symptoms and signs ever occurring in patients with SLE.

As medical knowledge of SLE has increased, the classification criteria of SLE has evolved to aid in the recognition of SLE. Although classification criteria have a prominent role in research studies to include or exclude study subjects, clinicians are certainly aware of these criteria. Clinicians often use the classification criteria to support a diagnosis of SLE in individual patients. **Table 2** shows how the SLE classification criteria evolved from 1971[13] to 1982[14] to 1997[15] to 2012[16] to 2019.[17]

Although SLE is the prototypical systemic autoimmune disease, there are other connective tissue disorders that can present with similar symptoms or overlap with SLE. When a person presents with multiple organ involvement, clinicians should consider

Table 1
Symptom and sign occurrence in systemic lupus erythematosus

Symptom or Sign	Percentage
Arthralgia	95
Neurologic	90
Fever >100°F (38°C)	90
Prolonged of extreme fatigue	81
Arthritis	80
Skin rashes	74
Anemia	71
Kidney involvement	50
Pleurisy and/or pericarditis	45
Malar rash	42
Photosensitivity	30
Hair loss	27
Blood clotting disorder	20
Raynaud phenomenon	17
Seizures	15
Mouth or nose ulcers	12

Adapted from The Lupus Initiative. Available at: https://thelupusinitiative.org/slides/pdf/PP_Overview_Supplementary_Materials.pdf, Accessed 28 February 2020.

Table 2
Lupus classification criteria evolving through the years

1982 Criteria[14]	1997 Update to 1982 Criteria[15]	2012 SLICC Criteria[16]	2019 Criteria[17]
Malar rash	Malar rash	Clinical criteria	Antinuclear antibodies
Discoid rash	Discoid rash	Acute cutaneous lupus	Fever
Photosensitivity	Photosensitivity	Chronic cutaneous lupus	Leukopenia
Oral ulcers	Oral ulcers	Oral ulcers	Thrombocytopenia
Arthritis	Arthritis	Nonscarring alopecia	Autoimmune hemolysis
Serositis	Serositis	Synovitis involving 2 or more joints, characterized by swelling or effusion	Delirium
Renal disorder	Renal disorder	Serositis	Psychosis
Neurologic disorder	Neurologic disorder	Renal	Seizure
Hematologic disorder	Hematologic disorder	Neurologic	Nonscarring alopecia
Immunologic disorder	Immunologic disorder (deleted "positive LE cell preparation" and added "positive finding of antiphospholipid antibodies" from 1982 criteria)	Hemolytic anemia	Oral ulcers
Antinuclear antibody	Antinuclear antibody	Leukopenia	Subacute cutaneous or discoid lupus
		Thrombocytopenia	Acute cutaneous lupus
		Immunologic criteria	Pleural or pericardial effusion
		Antinuclear antibody level higher than laboratory reference range	Acute pericarditis
		Anti-dsDNA antibody level higher than laboratory reference range	Joint involvement
		Anti-Smith antibody	Proteinuria >0.5 g/24 h

(continued on next page)

1982 Criteria[14]	1997 Update to 1982 Criteria[15]	2012 SLICC Criteria[16]	2019 Criteria[17]
		Antiphospholipid antibody	Class II or V lupus nephritis on renal biopsy according to ISN/RPS 2003 classification
		Low complement	Class III or IV lupus nephritis on renal biopsy according to ISN/RPS 2003 classification
		Direct Coombs test in the absence of hemolytic anemia	Positive antiphospholipid antibodies
			Low C3 OR low C4
			Low C3 AND low C4
			Anti-dsDNA antibodies or anti-Smith antibodies

Table 2 (continued)

Abbreviations: C3, complement 3; C4, complement 4; dsDNA, double-stranded DNA; ISN/RPS, International Society of Nephrology/Renal Pathology Society; SLICC, Systemic Lupus International Collaborating Clinics.

infections, malignancy, and autoimmune causes. A through history and physical coupled with a comprehensive review of systems aids the clinician as they consider the most appropriate diagnosis and treatment plan. **Box 1** includes a list of conditions that could be included in the differential diagnosis when a person presents when SLE is being considered.

It is important for clinicians to be constantly vigilant when patients present with symptoms to suggest systemic autoimmune conditions. One survey of patients with SLE asked these persons to identify the symptoms they experienced before and during the first year of their SLE diagnosis. Fatigue (89.4%), joint pain (86.7%), photosensitivity (79.4%), myalgia (76.1%), and skin rashes (70.5%) were the most commonly described symptoms before and during the first year of diagnosis. Fever (53.7%) and Raynaud (51.9%) were also described by more than half of these persons.[18]

It is evident that initial symptoms that often lead to an SLE diagnosis also occur with other rheumatic and nonrheumatic conditions. One study indicated that persons diagnosed with lupus, when compared with lupus-mimicking conditions, more often presented with unexplained fevers, weight loss, malar rash, photosensitivity, oral ulcers, and alopecia. Lupus-mimicking conditions more often presented with the following symptoms: Raynaud phenomenon, sicca symptoms, dysphagia, and fatigue.[19]

Although the cause of lupus is not currently known, some patients do present with systemic lupus-like symptoms as a result of their use of certain medications. When taking a drug that is believed to be the cause of lupus symptoms, this is called drug-induced lupus. Although many drugs have been believed to possibly be culprits,

---

Box 1
Conditions to consider in the SLE differential diagnosis

- Infection (bacterial and viral)
- Malignancy
- Rheumatoid arthritis
- Rhupus (an overlap syndrome including lupus and rheumatoid arthritis)
- Mixed connective tissue disease: an overlap condition with SLE, systemic sclerosis, and polymyositis features with a supporting (+) U1 ribonucleoprotein antibody
- Undifferentiated connective tissue disease
- Drug-induced lupus
- Sjögren syndrome
- Systemic sclerosis
- Vasculitis
- Behçet syndrome
- Polymyositis
- Dermatomyositis
- Adult Still disease
- Serum sickness
- Fibromyalgia
- Thrombotic thrombocytopenic purpura
- Multiple sclerosis

---

the following drugs are the most common causes of drug-induced lupus with category of risk provided: hydralazine (high risk), procainamide (high risk), isoniazid (moderate risk), minocycline (low risk), and more recently reported tumor necrosis factor-α inhibitors.[20]

Drug-induced lupus is often associated with the presence of histone antibodies. Those with drug-induced lupus may have systemic features, but do not typically have central nervous system or renal manifestations. When the offending drug agent causing drug-induced lupus is discontinued, the associated symptoms often resolve.

LABORATORY AND ANCILLARY TESTS

Together with a comprehensive history and physical examination, ancillary tests aid the practitioner in diagnosing and monitoring persons with SLE. In this section, we discuss laboratory studies to aid with diagnosis and monitoring of persons with SLE and the use of biopsy tissue samples for diagnostic and treatment determination purposes.

Laboratory

As the classification criteria indicate, SLE can potentially affect all cell lines. Leukopenia, lymphopenia, hemolytic anemia, and thrombocytopenia can occur with SLE. A complete blood count (CBC) with differential is a critical screening tool when SLE is suspected to look for deficiencies in all blood cell lines. The CBC should also be ordered periodically to monitor persons with known SLE to ensure that new hematologic disease manifestations have not occurred. The frequency of CBC ordering is based on disease activity, previous results, and current medications. When changes in CBC are noted, it is incumbent on the clinician to decide if the changes are related to disease causes, medication effects, or other non-SLE-related causes.

Serologic metabolic chemistry laboratory serves a role in the initial diagnostic recognition of SLE and the long-term monitoring of SLE. Of particular importance is renal function as indicated by the serum blood urea nitrogen measurement, the serum creatinine, and the serum albumin. These laboratory parameters should be monitored over time and compared with previous results to look for trends suggestive of kidney function deterioration. Hepatic function is also key to note. Other comorbid liver disease regardless of cause (infectious, structural, autoimmune, or otherwise) affect potential treatment options.

A urinalysis also serves a role in measuring renal function in SLE. When a urinalysis shows proteinuria, pyuria, hematuria, and/or cellular casts without a known cause, the clinician must search for the cause. If these results are seen in a patient with known or suspected systemic autoimmunity, further renal specific studies must be considered. When protein is noted on urinalysis, an albumin to creatinine ratio or a 24-hour urine collection for total protein and creatinine clearance is used to quantify the amount of proteinuria, which is important when considering SLE-related kidney disease and its treatment.

ANA is the most common laboratory study associated with SLE. There are multiple laboratory techniques used to identify ANA, but the American College of Rheumatology has published a position statement supporting the use of the immunofluorescence ANA test using Human Epithelial type 2 (HEp-2) substrate, as the gold standard for ANA testing.[21] This is the laboratory technique that provides a titer and pattern if ANA are detected.

It is also notable that ANA results are positive in other rheumatic and nonrheumatic conditions. **Box 2** lists some conditions also associated with ANAs and the usefulness of the ANA in the diagnosis.[22]

Like other laboratory studies, it must be recognized that the sensitivity and specificity of the ANA laboratory test for lupus is not 100%. A systematic review of the literature provides some insight to further understand the value of ANA titers and the relationship to sensitivity and specificity (**Table 3**).[23]

Depending on the titer result and the clinician's level of suspicion for the presence of SLE or another systemic autoimmune condition, additional, more specific autoantibodies laboratory are considered. **Table 4** lists some of the most common autoantibodies used to further clarify the diagnosis of SLE or other systemic autoimmune conditions.[24,25] As part of the American College of Rheumatology's Choosing Wisely efforts, the ordering of ANA subserologies should not be done without a positive ANA and clinical suspicion of "immune-mediated disease."[26] ANA and other autoantibodies should not be ordered without a high pretest probability and level of clinical suspicion for systemic autoimmune disease. An exception may occur with strong clinical suspicion for SLE but with a negative ANA in which testing for SS-A and SS-B are appropriate.

It is also notable that ANA and other ANA subserologies may be present before the onset of clinical disease.[27,28] If an ANA is found to be significantly positive without known clinical suspicion, a careful comprehensive multisystem history and physical examination looking for subtle autoimmune symptoms and signs should be performed, and if none are found, periodic follow-up with attention to possible evolving autoimmune features is advisable.

Box 2
Conditions associated with a (+) ANA and its diagnostic usefulness

ANA very useful
  Systemic lupus erythematosus
  Systemic sclerosis

ANA somewhat useful
  Sjögren syndrome
  Polymyositis
  Dermatomyositis

ANA very useful for monitoring or prognosis
  Juvenile chronic arthritis
  Raynaud phenomenon

ANA critical for diagnosis
  Drug-induced lupus
  Mixed connective tissue disease
  Autoimmune hepatitis

ANA not useful for diagnosis, monitoring, or prognosis
  Rheumatoid arthritis
  Multiple sclerosis
  Thyroid disease
  Infectious disease
  Idiopathic thrombocytopenic purpura
  Fibromyalgia

From Solomon DH, Kavanaugh AJ, Schur P, et al., Evidence-based guidelines for the use of immunologic tests: antinuclear antibody testing. Arthritis Rheu. 2002; 47(4): 434-444; with permission.

Biopsy

Skin and kidney are the most common tissues biopsied for SLE diagnostic purposes. In this article we briefly provide an overview of renal biopsy in the setting of SLE.

The kidney is a target organ for SLE activity. Monitoring renal function through the use of laboratory and urinalysis is of vital importance to recognize and prevent morbidity and mortality associated with lupus nephritis. When the following are noted on screening laboratory studies, a kidney biopsy should be considered: increasing serum creatinine without alternative explanation, proteinuria of greater than or equal to 1 g/24 hour, or greater than or equal to 0.5 g/24 hour plus hematuria or cellular casts.[29] Additionally laboratory studies, such as double-stranded DNA and complements (C3, C4, and CH50), may also be used to evaluate lupus nephritis disease activity. Double-stranded DNA and complements should be compared with a patient's baseline levels. If a renal biopsy is determined to be indicated, the results can assist in guiding the clinician to specific treatment targeted toward the kidney. **Table 5** contains a summary of potential renal biopsy results and associated clinical manifestations.[29]

TREATMENT
Nonpharmacologic

There are numerous nonmedicine approaches that should be taken to ensure best outcomes for persons with SLE. Instructing and reminding patients and their support persons of these options should occur frequently.

Table 3 Sensitivities and specificities of ANA titers when diagnosing SLE		
Titer	Sensitivity (%)	Specificity (%)
1:40	98.4	66.9
1:80	97.8	74.7
1:160	95.8	86.2
1:320	86.0	96.6

Adapted from Leuchten N, Hoyer A, Brinks R, et al. Performance of antinuclear antibodies for classifying systemic lupus erythematosus: a systematic literature review and meta-regression of diagnostic data. Arthritis Care Res. 2018; 70(3):428-438; with permission.

Sun avoidance or protection is key so as to avoid cutaneous or systemic SLE exacerbations. Sunscreens and protective clothing and cosmetics are used to assist with sun protection.

Monitoring and controlling modifiable risk factors, such as weight, blood pressure, and lipids, must occur. Cardiovascular disease risk is greatly increased in patients with lupus as in other systemic inflammatory diseases, including in populations of patients not otherwise associated with high cardiovascular risk, such as young women. Clear communication among a person's health care team should occur to ensure that these features are being addressed.

Patients with SLE often are required to take corticosteroids at some point in their health journey. The clinician and the patients with SLE must be cognizant of their bone health status. Using corticosteroids at the lowest dose and for the shortest period of time is recommended. Weight-bearing activity and calcium with vitamin D supplementation should be encouraged.

Age-appropriate, killed vaccinations should be provided to patients with SLE. If a patient with SLE on immunosuppressive agents, including corticosteroids, live vaccinations should generally be avoided.

Steps to prevent disease flare or progression, such as infection avoidance measures, avoiding medications that may worsen renal function, and taking preventative

Table 4 Autoantibodies in SLE		
Antibodies	Prevalence (%)[25]	Clinical Associations
ANA		Nonspecific
Anti-dsDNA	70–80	Nephritis
Anti-Sm	10–30	Nonspecific
Anti-RNP		Arthritis, myositis, lung disease
Anti-SS-A	30–40	Dry eyes/mouth, SCLE, neonatal lupus, photosensitivity
Anti-SS-B	15–20	Same as SS-A
Antiphospholipid	20–30	Clotting diathesis

From The Lupus Initiative. Systemic Lupus Erythematosus Overview: Clinical Presentation, pathophysiology, and therapeutic strategies over the course of the disease. American College of Rheuamtology. https://thelupusinitiative.org/slides/pdf/PP_Overview.pdf. Accessed 03 March 2020.

Table 5
International Society of Nephrology and the Renal Pathology Society classification of renal biopsies

Class	Clinical Manifestations
I: minimal mesangial	None
II: mesangial proliferative	Microscopic hematuria ± proteinuria; rare hypertension
III: focal proliferative	Hematuria and proteinuria ± hypertension, decreased glomerular filtration rate, or nephrotic syndrome
IV: diffuse proliferative	Hematuria, proteinuria (frequently nephrotic), cellular casts, and generally decreased glomerular filtration rate; hypertension is common; hypocomplementemia and elevated dsDNA also seen frequently
V: membranous	Extensive proteinuria with minimal hematuria or renal function abnormalities
VI: advanced sclerosing	Chronic kidney disease

Abbreviations: dsDNA, double-stranded DNA; RNP, ribonucleoprotein; Sm, Smith; SS-A, Sjögren syndrome related antigen A; SS-B, Sjögren syndrome related antigen B.

From Zell J, Griffith M. Systemic Lupus Erythematosus. In: West SG, Kolfenbach J. Rheumatology Secrets. 4th Edition. Philadelphia: Elsevier; 2020: 131-151; with permission.

steps to avoid clots in patients with SLE is encouraged. Thrombosis risk is higher in patients with SLE compared with the general population.

When a patient with SLE presents with symptoms, the clinician must maintain an open mind and differential diagnosis so as not to contribute, when inappropriate, the presenting symptoms solely to SLE.

Pharmacologic

A handful of medications (aspirin [1948], prednisone [1950s], hydroxychloroquine [1955], and most recently belimumab [2011]) have received a Food and Drug Administration indication for the treatment of SLE. Although many other medications (including immunosuppressive medications) are used to treat lupus, the paucity of Food and Drug Administration–approved medications suggests the importance of ongoing scientific investigation to better understand the pathophysiology and optimal pharmacologic treatment options. Some of the immunosuppressive medications used to treat SLE include, but are not limited to, the following: methotrexate, leflunomide, azathioprine, cyclophosphamide, and mycophenolate mofetil. The choice of which pharmacologic treatment is based on the person's SLE disease manifestations and their comorbidities. Each of these medications are powerful yet can provide benefit. Vigilant adherence to monitoring through laboratory and follow-up visits with a health care provider are essential. A further discussion regarding these treatment options, except for hydroxychloroquine (discussed next), is beyond the scope of this article.

Hydroxychloroquine has been used for more than half a century and is recognized for its cutaneous,[30] articular,[31] hematologic,[32] and renal (together with other immunosuppressive)[33,34] benefits. Hydroxychloroquine is generally well tolerated and should be recommended for most persons with SLE. The current recommended dose is less than or equal to 5 mg/kg real weight/d. Exceeding 400 mg/d is not recommended. The American Academy of Ophthalmology recommends an initial fundus examination to rule out retinopathy, and then annual examination after the patient has taken hydroxychloroquine for 5 years. The preferred screening test is an automated visual field plus spectral-domain optical coherence tomography.[35]

SUMMARY

SLE is a complex disease that requires a multidisciplinary team to achieve best patient outcomes. Health care providers, including physician assistants, in numerous medical specialties (eg, primary care, rheumatology, dermatology, nephrology, neurology, pulmonology, cardiology) may participate on an individual's health care team based on disease manifestations. Other health professionals are also key. Being a chronic condition, the patient and the provider have the opportunity to work together to choose best treatment and monitoring approaches for best outcomes.

Advances have been made in the understanding of the pathophysiology, diagnosis, and treatment of SLE. Additional discovery awaits.

CLINICS CARE POINTS

- The Systemic Lupus Erythematosus (SLE) classification criteria has evolved over years and include multiple systemic manifestations of SLE.
- The immunofluorescence ANA laboratory testing technique is the gold standard for ANA laboratory testing.
- Hydroxychloroquine should be included as a treatment option for most persons with SLE.

ACKNOWLEDGEMENTS

Special thanks to Dr Victor M. McMillan for assisting in the writing of this article by providing constructive feedback.

DISCLOSURE

No financial relationships to disclose.

REFERENCES

1. Blotzer JW. Systemic lupus erythematosus, I: historical aspects. Md State Med J 1983;32:439–41.
2. Holubar K. Terminology and iconography of lupus erythematosus: a historical vignette. Am J Dermatopathol 1980;2:239–42.
3. Lahita RG. Systemic lupus erythematosus. New York: John Wiley and Sons; 1987.
4. Osler W. On the visceral complications of erythema exudativum multiforme. Am J Med Sci 1895;110:629–46.
5. Hargraves MM. Discovery of the LE cell and its morphology. Mayo Clin Proc 1969;44:579–99.
6. Rees F, Doherty M, Grainge MJ, et al. The worldwide incidence and prevalence systemic lupus erythematosus: a systematic review of epidemiological studies. Rheumatology (Oxford) 2017;56(11):1945–61.
7. Somers EC, Marder W, Cagnoli P, et al. Population-based incidence and prevalence of systemic lupus erythematosus: the Michigan lupus epidemiology and surveillance program. Arthritis Rheumatol 2014;66(2):369–78.

8. Lim SS, Bayakly AR, Helmick CG, et al. The incidence and prevalence of systemic lupus erythematosus, 2002–2004: the Georgia lupus registry. Arthritis Rheumatol 2014;66(2):357–68.

9. Ferucci ED, Johnston JM, Gaddy JR, et al. Prevalence and incidence of systemic lupus erythematosus in a population-based registry of American Indian and Alaska native people, 2007–2009. Arthritis Rheumatol 2014;66(9):2494–502.

10. Dall'Era M, Cisternas MG, Snipes K, et al. The incidence and prevalence of systemic lupus erythematosus in San Francisco County, California: the California lupus surveillance project. Arthritis Rheumatol 2017;69(10):1996–2005.

11. Izmirly PM, Wan I, Sahl S, et al. The incidence and prevalence of systemic lupus erythematosus in New York County (Manhattan), New York: the Manhattan lupus surveillance program. Arthritis Rheumatol 2017;69(10):2006–17.

12. Riveros Frutos A, Casas I, Rua-Figueroa I, et al. Systemic lupus erythematosus in Spanish males: a study of the Spanish rheumatology society lupus registry (REL-ESSER) cohort. Lupus 2017;(7):698–706.

13. Cohen AS, Reynolds WE, Franklin EC, et al. Preliminary criteria for the classification of systemic lupus erythematosus. Bull Rheum Dis 1971;21:643–8.

14. Tan EM, Cohen AS, Fries JF, et al. The 1982 revised criteria for the classification of systemic lupus erythematosus. Arthritis Rheumatol 1982;25:1271–7.

15. Hochberg MC. Updating the American College of Rheumatology revised criteria for the classification of systemic lupus erythematosus [letter]. Arthritis Rheumatol 1997;40:1725.

16. Petri M, Orbai AM, Alarcon GS, et al. Derivation and validation of Systemic Lupus International Collaborating Clinics classification criteria for systemic lupus erythematosus. Arthritis Rheumatol 2012;64(8):2677–86.

17. Aringer M, Costenbader K, Daikh D, et al. 2019 European League Against Rheumatism/American College of Rheumatology classification criteria for systemic lupus erythematosus. Arthritis Rheumatol 2019;71(9):1400–12.

18. Leuchten N, Milke B, Winkler-Rohlfing B, et al. Early symptoms of systemic lupus erythematosus (SLE) recalled by 339 SLE patients. Lupus 2018;27:1431–6.

19. Mosca M, Costenbader KH, Johnson SR, et al. How do patients with newly diagnosed systemic lupus erythematosus present? A multicenter cohort of early systemic lupus erythematosus to inform the development of new classification criteria. Arthritis Rheumatol 2019;71(1):91–8.

20. Hea Y, Sawalhaa AH. Drug-induced lupus erythematosus: an update on drugs and mechanisms. Curr Opin Rheumatol 2018;30:490–7.

21. American College of Rheumatology. Methodology of testing for antinuclear antibodies. American College of Rheumatology. 2015. Available at: https://www.rheumatology.org/Portals/0/Files/Methodology%20of%20Testing%20Antinuclear%20Antibodies%20Position%20Statement.pdf. Accessed February 28, 2020.

22. Solomon DH, Kavanaugh AJ, Schur P, et al. Evidence-based guidelines for the use of immunologic tests: antinuclear antibody testing. Arthritis Rheumatol 2002;47(4):434–44.

23. Leuchten N, Hoyer A, Brinks R, et al. Performance of antinuclear antibodies for classifying systemic lupus erythematosus: a systematic literature review and meta-regression of diagnostic data. Arthritis Care Res 2018;70(3):428–38.

24. The Lupus Initiative. Systemic lupus erythematosus overview: clinical presentation, pathophysiology, and therapeutic strategies over the course of the disease. American College of Rheumatology. Available at: https://thelupusinitiative.org/slides/pdf/PP_Overview.pdf. Accessed March 03, 2020.

25. Rahman A, Isenberg DA. Systemic lupus erythematosus. N Engl J Med 2008; 358(9):929–39.
26. Yazdany J, Schmajuk A, Robbins M, et al. Choosing wisely: the American College of Rheumatology's top 5 list of things physicians and patients should question. Arthritis Care Res 2013;65(3):329–39.
27. Arbuckle MR, McClain MT, Rubertone MV, et al. Development of autoantibodies before the clinical onset of systemic lupus erythematosus. N Engl J Med 2003; 349(16):1526–33.
28. Heinlen LD, McClain MT, Merrill J, et al. Clinical criteria for systemic lupus erythematosus precede diagnosis, and associated autoantibodies are present before clinical symptoms. Arthritis Rheumatol 2007;56:2344–51.
29. Zell J, Griffith M. Systemic lupus erythematosus. In: West SG, Kolfenbach J, editors. Rheumatology secrets. 4th edition. Philadelphia: Elsevier; 2020. p. 131–51.
30. Pons-Estel GJ, Alarcón GS, González LA, et al. Possible protective effect of hydroxychloroquine on delaying the occurrence of integument damage in lupus: LXXI, data from a multiethnic cohort. Arthritis Care Res 2010;62:393–400.
31. Williams HJ, Egger MJ, Singer JZ, et al. Comparison of hydroxychloroquine and placebo in the treatment of the arthropathy of mild systemic lupus erythematosus. J Rheumatol 1994;21:1457–62.
32. Arnal C, Piette JC, Léone J, et al. Treatment of severe immune thrombocytopenia associated with systemic lupus erythematosus: 59 cases. J Rheumatol 2002;29: 75–83.
33. Pons-Estel GJ, Alarcón GS, McGwin G, et al. Protective effect of hydroxychloroquine on renal damage in patients with lupus nephritis: LXV, data from a multiethnic US cohort. Arthritis Rheumatol 2009;61:830–9.
34. Kasitanon N, Fine DM, Haas M, et al. Hydroxychloroquine use predicts complete renal remission within 12 months among patients treated with mycophenolate mofetil therapy for membranous lupus nephritis. Lupus 2006;15:366–70.
35. Marmor MF, Kellner U, Tai TY, et al. American Academy of Ophthalmology, recommendations of screening for chloroquine and hydroxychloroquine retinopathy (2016 revision). Ophthalmology 2016;123:1386–94.

Gout and Other Crystal Arthritides

Joan McTigue, PA-C, MS

KEYWORDS

- Gout • Calcium phosphate deposition disease • Basic calcium deposition disease

KEY POINTS

- In contrast with calcium containing crystals, gout is caused by crystalline deposits of monosodium urate.
- The body burden of monosodium urate crystals can be greatly decreased, if not eliminated, by urate-lowering medications.
- Although there is no elimination therapy for excess deposits of calcium crystals, both types of crystalline arthritis can be very inflammatory and very painful.
- Looking forward, many enthusiastic national and international research laboratories are investigating the genetic, molecular, and biochemical processes of crystalline arthropathies with steady progress toward therapies.

AN OVERVIEW OF CRYSTAL-INDUCED ARTHROPATHIES

As populations live longer, osteoarthritis and crystal deposition disorders become more prevalent, affecting both articular and periarticular tissues.[1] Crystalline arthritis can be acute or chronic, involving 1, a few, or multiple joints. They often develop in joints afflicted by trauma or degenerative arthritis. In addition, crystal deposition can incidentally be seen in images of joints and periarticular structures without the development of symptoms. When symptomatic, these disorders are inflammatory conditions. The inflammation develops when components of the innate immune system develop activating interaction between macrophages and crystals. These are not autoimmune conditions.[2] It is important to distinguish the arthritis of crystal deposition from infection, trauma, and degenerative arthritis (**Table 1**). Be aware that they can coexist.

GOUT

Gout is the classic crystal-induced inflammatory arthritis clinically well-characterized by ancient and modern writers. It has become the most common inflammatory arthritis in the United States. By the last National Health and Nutrition Examination Survey

Division of Rheumatology, VA Medical Center and University of Florida, Gainesville, FL, USA
E-mail address: jcmctigue@gmail.com

Physician Assist Clin 6 (2021) 75–88
https://doi.org/10.1016/j.cpha.2020.09.008
2405-7991/21/Published by Elsevier Inc.

physicianassistant.theclinics.com

Table 1 An overview of crystal type and crystal deposition disorders	
Crystal Type	**Disorder**
Monosodium urate	Gout
Calcium pyrophosphate dihydrate	Calcium pyrophosphate deposition disease, or pseudogout
Basic calcium phosphate	
Intra-articular deposits	Acute synovitis and destructive arthropathy
Periarticular deposits	Acute calcific periarthritis, periarticular pain

report, in the United States, there are approximately 9 million sufferers. Gout can develop in a younger person with a strong family history, but the average age of onset is approximately 55 years in men. Gout occurs as well in females, largely in postmenopausal women. Estrogen is protective against hyperuricemia. That benefit disappears after estrogen levels wane.[3]

Ethnic and race variables exist regarding prevalence. In the Asian-Pacific regions, gout is far more common than in the United States. Family history is a strong contributor in all groups.[4]

Gout is best conceptualized as a disease of urate burden. This concept can be taught to patients, just as we explain the burden of high cholesterol in coronary artery disease. Gout results from tissue deposition of plasma monosodium urate (MSU), which crystalizes in joints and soft tissue when elevated beyond its natural point of solubility. Humans lack the enzyme uricase, which oxidizes insoluble uric acid to the much more soluble and easily excretable allantoin. Uric acid is eliminated in small part by the gut, but largely by the kidney. Its relative insolubility makes renal uric acid excretion subject to easy perturbation, leading to hyperuricemia and crystallization when present in excess.[5]

Given the right circumstances, these uric acid crystal deposits can beget flares of rapid onset acute monoarticular (and, in time, polyarticular) inflammatory arthritis. Not all persons with hyperuricemia develop gout. However, the higher the serum uric acid, the more likely gout will develop, particularly in those with strong family histories of gout.[5]

Uric acid (urate) is a natural product of purine metabolism. Purines bases are derived largely from endogenous cellular sources as they naturally break down. Our diets contain sources of purines as well. Dietary sources contribute far less to the body urate pool than do endogenous sources. It is important to stress this concept. Clinicians tend to overemphasize diet. Patients can become fixated on dietary change as the primary route to lowering plasma uric acid level.

Uric acid stays soluble in plasma up to 6.8 mg/dL and, as stated elsewhere in this article, is largely excreted by the kidneys. Once chronically above the level of solubility, hyperuricemia is the biochemical state and from hyperuricemia can develop gout. Biochemical hyperuricemia is best defined as a plasma uric acid level of 6.8 mg/dL or higher. However, laboratory-generated reference ranges are based on averages of plasma uric acid in a given population. They are not relevant to the biochemical level at which crystals and therefore gout symptoms develop. Thus, anyone with a plasma uric acid consistently greater than 6.8 mg/dL may be at risk for the development of gout.

Hyperuricemia is the metabolic underpinning of gout. It may also play a deleterious role in other disorders, such as the development of renal stones. Research in recent years has shown us that hyperuricemia worsens other metabolic disorders as well.

It is important to stress not all patients with hyperuricemia develop gout. The 5-year cumulative incidence of gout in patients with a serum urate of greater than 7 mg/dL is approximately 20%. However, the cumulative incidence with a urate of greater than 9.0 mg/dL increases to approximately 60%.

As our diets became purine richer, as renal clearance decreased, and as certain medication use (diuretics and transplant rejection agents in particular) grew, increased numbers of adults in the United States and abroad now have serum urate values at or above the level of solubility.[6]

Causes of Hyperuricemia

In humans, uric acid can be overproduced, underexcreted, or both. Overproduction accounts for approximately 10% of hyperuricemia and is caused by inherited disorders of purine synthesis, as seen in juvenile or early-onset gout. Rapid cell turnover caused by illnesses such as tumor lysis syndrome, which can accompany chemotherapy or leukemias, can cause an overproduction of purines. Thankfully, current chemotherapy regimens cause far less tumor lysis syndrome than in decades past. Last, excessive dietary purine intake such as binge drinking especially beer or over eating high purine shell foods can tip into excessive production of purines.

Underexcretion by the kidney causes most cases of hyperuricemia. A number of conditions alter kidney uric acid excretion. These include

- Renal insufficiency from diabetes or hypertension.
- Lactic acidosis and ketoacidosis.
- Diuretic and transplant rejection medication use.
- Dehydration.
- Rare, but still seen, is overexposure to lead.

Pathogenesis of Gout

Once the limit of solubility (6.8 mg/dL) is exceeded, plasma uric acid can crystallize as a monosodium salt in synovial tissue, on the surface of cartilage, and in joint fluid. Over time the crystals can deposit in soft tissue. Lumps called tophi form. Clusters of uric acid can be seen in other tissues as well, for example, urate stones in the kidneys.

Under certain circumstances, urate crystals activate synovial resident inflammatory cells, which initiates the acute gouty process. This topic is a keen area of research and the mechanisms are being worked out. At the cellular level, a fundamental mechanism of crystal-induced inflammation seems to be engagement of crystals with the innate immune system via pattern recognition receptors on mononuclear phagocytes. From that event, the innate immune system is rapidly activated and a complex cascade of inflammation is quickly amplified.

Neutrophil migration into the joint seems to be the most important event driving the severe inflammatory process that a gout flare becomes. Likewise, the turn off process is under active investigation. Unlike other inflammatory arthritides like rheumatoid arthritis, gout is, at first, a self-limiting process (**Fig. 1**). During these events, proinflammatory cytokines (especially IL-1) in the joint enter the circulation and account for the systemic features such as fever, chills, and elevated inflammatory markers experienced by many gout flare sufferers. This condition can be hard to distinguish clinically from a septic joint.

Acute Gout: Clinical Presentation

Acute gout is joint based. An acute attack of rapid onset, intense pain—usually in lower extremity joints—develops after recent trauma, dietary indiscretion,

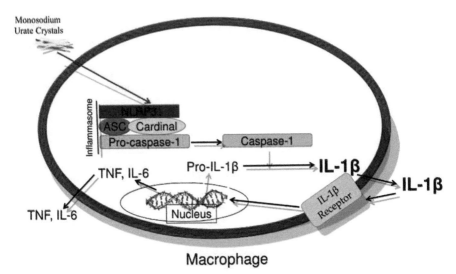

Fig. 1. The inflammasome, a central mediator of gout inflammation. Inflammasomes are key signaling platforms within various immune system cells that detect pathogenic microorganisms and nonsterile stressors such as crystals, which then activate highly proinflammatory cytokines. TNF, tumor necrosis factor. (*Courtesy of* NL Edwards, MD.)

postoperative bed rest, dehydration, or acidosis. It often begins in the night with full symptoms apparent in the morning. Twinges of discomfort progress to severe pain over 8 to 10 hours with mounting clinical evidence of intense synovitis—that is, the red, hot swollen joint. Gout commonly effects the great toe (podagra). It is not unusual to affect the knee, mid foot, wrist, and elbow. There are rare reports in the spine (**Fig. 2**).[7]

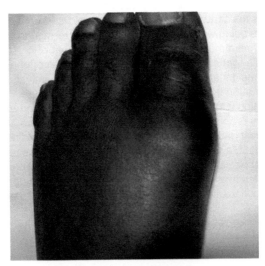

Fig. 2. Great toe with the acute inflammation of gout.

Fevers and chills accompany acute gout in one-third of gout flares owing to the cytokine release described elsewhere in this article. Interestingly, serum urate levels decrease during acute gout, often resulting temporarily in a falsely normal laboratory value. Weight bearing or wearing restrictive clothes like a shoe is often impossible with the acutely inflamed joint. Untreated or suboptimally treated gout flares last for 4 to 8 days in the early phases and up to 2 weeks as time passes. The body's urate burden continues to increase if not modified by urate-lowering therapy.

Advanced Gout

With time (decades usually) of sustained untreated hyperuricemia, gout can become polyarticular. Renal stones occur in 25% of gouty patients. Subcutaneous tophi can develop over extensor surfaces. These are firm nodules of urate crystals surrounded by a foreign body granuloma. Chronic tophaceous gout can develop within the joints causing erosions and deformity[8] (Fig. 3).

Making the Diagnosis

Presumed gout is thought of as a soft but generally accurate diagnosis based on a history of recurrent rapid onset, very hot, painful monoarthritis in the background setting of hyperuricemia. Family history is often a factor, as is alcohol abuse.

Gout has an excellent clinical response to early use of anti-inflammatory agents (nonsteroidal anti-inflammatory drugs, colchicine, corticosteroids). However, the longer the flare goes on without anti-inflammatory therapy, the harder it is to abort.

Definitive gout as a diagnosis rests on microscopically proven MSU crystals seen in synovial fluid aspirated from an acute presentation or the presence of tophi or characteristic imaging consistent with gout. Ultrasound examination, MRI, and dual imaging computed tomography scans are far more sensitive than plain films, but are far less quickly available. Erosive bone damage advanced enough to be seen on plain films are usually a late finding. Early flares of gout have no radiographic findings other than soft tissue swelling.

In the acute attack, the gold standard evidence is intracellular, needle-shaped crystals with a strong negative birefringence seen on polarizing microscopy. However, aspirating and viewing synovial fluid is not often feasible in many clinical settings[8] (Fig. 4).

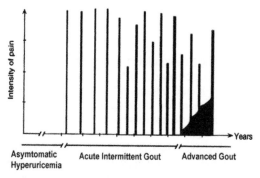

Fig. 3. At first, gout flares are intermittent. If untreated, over time they come more frequently. Then chronic painful synovitis develops as well as joint deformities and tophaceous deposits. (*From* Edwards NL. Gout. In: Klippel JH, Stone JH, Crofford LJ, et al. (eds) Primer on the Rheumatic Diseases. Springer, New York, NY. https://doi.org/10.1007/978-0-387-68566-3_12; with permission.)

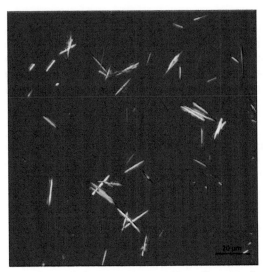

Fig. 4. Gout crystals seen by a polarizing microscope. The yellow, needle-shaped objects are the gout crystals. (*From* Dalbeth N, Merriman TR, Stamp LK. Gout. Lancet. 2016;388(10055):2039-2052. https://doi.org/10.1016/S0140-6736(16)00346-9; Reprinted with permission of Elsevier.)

Laboratory Findings

An elevated synovial fluid white blood cell count is noted in most infectious causes of a hot joint, as well as in inflammatory crystal-induced arthritis. Crystals observed in synovial fluid do not rule out infection. Only culture does. Elevated sedimentation rates (often impressive) are often seen in acute gout but have no specificity. When able to aspirate a joint, always send the aspirated synovial fluid to a laboratory. Order the 3 Cs—cell count, culture, and crystal analysis—under a polarizing light microscope. Be sure your laboratory uses this microscopic technique when looking for crystals. The plasma urate level is often falsely lower during a gout flare. Do not rely on a uric acid drawn during a gout flare to reflect the true plasma uric acid level. It must be checked in a nonflare state. Glucose, lipids, and creatinine levels should be looked at as well. They are diseases associated with gout. Hyperuricemia along with the metabolic syndrome is not at all unusual.[9]

Radiographic Findings

Assess bone and joint damage using plain radiographs although, as mentioned elsewhere in this article, in early cases of gout all that might be noted is soft tissue swelling. The emerging role of office-based ultrasound examination is an important development. Criteria are in development for validated use of this imagining tool.

Early inflammatory processes do not destroy joints. Yet, in time, they all do. Repeat inflammation in joints from sources such as rheumatoid arthritis, crystal-induced arthritis, and infection all cause destructive changes leading to joint deformities. Loss of function is common in advanced gout. This condition largely comes when early gout is untreated or undertreated. Treating repeat gout flares without treating the cause (hyperuricemia) by lowering uric acid levels to a target leads to joint destruction and eventually deformities.

Classic mid to late stage radiographic findings include overhanging edges and asymmetric destruction. Ultrasound examination and dual energy computed tomography imaging are emerging as very useful modalities to establish an earlier diagnosis, before joint destruction takes place. In-office ultrasound examination is becoming a point-of-care technology among rheumatologists.

Treatment of the Acute Flare

The goal is rapid relief of pain and inflammation. Acute gout will respond to the following therapies especially if started within the first 24 to 36 hours of the attack.

Nonsteroidal anti-inflammatory drugs—Most commonly used but at higher than usual doses

Colchicine—Two tablets of colchicine 0.6 mg at once and a third tablet 1 hour later. Then twice daily dosing until the flare is gone. There is no place for older colchicine regimens, although many patients remember them well.

Corticosteroids—Can be used orally (eg, a dose Pak), intramuscularly (80–120 mg IM of depomedrol or other equivalent IM steroid), or intra-articular therapy after aspiration.

Biologic-based therapies target the drivers of the immune response described elsewhere in this article; for example, anakinra 100 mg subcutaneous is an IL-1 inhibitor. IL-1 is the key cytokine in gout flares. Anakinra is well-tolerated and aborts flares quickly. It is not approved by the US Food and Drug Administration for acute gout but its use is becoming more common, especially in the hospitalized patient with a gout flare and comorbid contraindications to other therapies. It also works well for a patient whose flare has been untreated for several days.[8]

Best Practice Long Game: Urate-Lowering Therapy and Flare Back Prophylaxis

Treating pain is 1 side of the gout equation. The other side of the gout equation is maintaining patient in a symptom-free state while decreasing serum urate to less than 6.0 mg/dL, which is the target level. It is best to be even lower in the tophaceous patient or a patient with established erosive changes seen on imagining. They have a larger urate burden, which will take longer to reduce unless the uric acid gets in the range of 3 to 5 mg/dL[8] (**Fig. 5**).

Opinions differ on when to begin urate-lowering medication.[10] Guidelines differ. Most Rheumatologist follow the current American College of Rheumatology

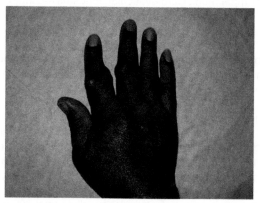

Fig. 5. A tophus in the second proximal interphalangeal joint. They can be seen in the toes, knees, fingers, wrists, elbows, and ears not uncommonly in advanced cases of poorly treated gout. (*Courtesy of* NL Edwards, MD.)

guideline.[11] On the basis of Level A evidence, the American College of Rheumatology guideline recommends "any patient with an established diagnosis of gouty arthritis and tophus/tophi or those with frequent attacks (>2 per year) be started on [urate-lowering therapy]." There is level C evidence in those recommendations for starting patients with gout with "[chronic kidney disease] stage 2 or worse plus those with past urolithiasis" on urate-lowering therapy. A treat to target approach was endorsed. Level A evidence endorsed "initiate concomitant pharmacologic anti-inflammatory gout attack prophylaxis when starting[urate-lowering therapy]."

Maintenance anti-inflammatory therapy with daily low-dose nonsteroidal anti-inflammatory drugs or colchicine 0.6 mg 2 to 4 times per day is recommended until the goal is met for 4 to 6 months. Occasionally, a low-dose steroid (prednisone 5–7.5 mg/d) is the safest approach. A flare-free patient with uric acid levels at target is the goal. In addition, patients should keep on hand medication to treat a flare. Urate-lowering therapy is not stopped during a gout flare.

Urate-lowering therapy in most patients with gout requires a lifelong commitment to therapy. There are several pharmacologic mechanisms to lower uric acid. Uric acid is rarely lowered sufficiently by dietary changes alone. Such changes should be encouraged, especially in heavy drinkers. However, practical experience shows dietary changes rarely induce changes in the plasma uric acid of more than 1 mg/dL. In most patients with gout, that is far from target.

Allopurinol is a xanthine oxidase inhibitor. It is currently the most commonly used urate-lowering therapy available to achieve uric acid levels of less than 6.0 mg/dL. It is inexpensive. When dosed at 50 to 300 mg, it is taken in a single daily dose. At doses of more than 600 mg/d, splitting the dose into a morning and evening dose is helpful. The maximal dose per the US Food and Drug Administration is 800 mg/d. However, it often takes a higher dose to reach target.[12]

Caution should be taken in those with renal or hepatic insufficiency. Begin at 50 mg/d in those individuals. Slowly titrate up in 3 intervals. Allopurinol is not renally dosed, however. Go low, go slow, and get to the right dose. The right dose is the dose that keeps the uric acid under 6.0 mg. The patient must report any signs of hypersensitivity at once, especially rash, and be rapidly evaluated for allopurinol hypersensitivity syndrome. In persons whose renal or hepatic function is normal, begin allopurinol at 100 mg/d and titrate up from there in the same intervals.

Febuxostat (Uloric) a newer xanthine oxidase inhibitor, is well-tolerated and especially useful in renal impairment. Cardiovascular concerns recently came from CARES, a trial of this agent versus allopurinol in those with cardiac disease.[13] The primary end point of the trial was the occurrence of a major adverse cardiovascular event in either treatment group. The secondary end points were the individual major adverse cardiovascular event components (cardiovascular death, nonfatal myocardial infarction, nonfatal stroke, and unstable angina requiring urgent revascularization). All-cause mortality was also analyzed. The primary end point of the trial was not significantly different between febuxostat (10.8%) and allopurinol (10.4%). However, within the secondary end points, cardiovascular death did show a significant difference between febuxostat (4.3%) and allopurinol (3.2%). Many questions remain about the meaning of the CARES study. To date, no physiologic mechanism has been detected. A larger trial will be published in 2020 or 2021, which will shed more light on this issue.

Begin febuxostat at 40 mg. As with use of allopurinol, recheck uric acid around 3 weeks into therapy and titrate the dose up to achieve the target. There is a once a day 80 mg dose as well. In terms of equivalency, allopurinol 300 mg and febuxostat 40 mg are roughly equivalent. There does not seem to be cross-allergies between these 2 therapies.[13]

An additional urate-lowering therapy includes probenecid, a uricosuric agent. That mode of action facilitates uric acid handling in the kidney. It requires dosing 2 to 3 times per day and loses effect as renal function declines. Adequate hydration a must. Probenecid is not used in those with a history of renal stones or known overproducers of uric acid. It can be add-on therapy to allopurinol or febuxostat.

Pegloticase (Krystexxa) is a major addition to the armamentarium of urate-lowering agents. It is infusible uricase, the enzyme humans lack to easily excrete uric acid. It has dramatic effect on tophi reduction. As a result, meaningful function to affected joints can be restored. There may be infusion reactions to this agent, but strategies to blunt infusion reactions have been developed. It can be infused on an outpatient basis in infusion offices or centers. Most generalists refer those who might be candidates for this therapy to a specialist (**Box 1**).

Lifestyle Changes

Encourage understanding gout as a disease of urate burden in an informative, nonjudgmental way. The analogy that consistently elevated glucose levels lead to diabetes or consistently high cholesterol levels can cause serious heart disease are useful analogies. These are fairly well-entrenched understandings in the general population.

Nonpharmacologic approaches to urate lowering are empowering. Older low-purine diets are not necessary and are often feel punitive to patients. Very high purine foods and drinks are listed in **Box 2**. As with many chronic conditions, a Mediterranean diet is an excellent dietary plan. It is tasty, healthful, and does not require special food avoidances.

Often, patients with gout are heavy drinkers, especially beer. It is a challenge to get them to limit alcohol. Counseling can be very useful. Weight management, high fructose corn syrup elimination, and the management of comorbidities are also essential. Data emerge regularly supporting a direct role of uric acid in various nonarticular diseases, including renal disease, hypertension, obesity, and, perhaps, cardiovascular disease as well.[9]

Poor health literacy is a major impediment to successful gout management. Nonjudgmental understanding is essential. Gout is not a disease of poor will power or an indulgent lifestyle, but is one of urate burden. With persistence and support, it can be managed successfully. Gouteducation.org is a very useful tool for patients and clinicians. They offer both on-line and written materials without cost.

Box 1
Summary

Begin with allopurinol at 100 mg or febuxostat at 40 mg/d. Begin with allopurinol 50 mg or febuxostat 20 mg in those with severe kidney impairment. Hold the dose there for 3 weeks.

Repeat a serum uric acid level then titrate the dose up by 3-week intervals until the treatment target is achieved. A treat-to-target approach is necessary and, like cholesterol levels, can easily be understood by clinicians and patients.

Achieve a uric acid of less than 6.0 mg/dL in most patients and lower in the tophaceous individual or those with imaging changes already established. They carry a higher urate burden and require a lower target uric acid such as 3 to 5 mg/dL.

Keep anti-inflammatory agents on board until the patient is at the uric acid target and is flare free. Do not stop urate-lowering therapy during a gout flare.

Refer the difficult-to-treat patients to a specialist. Consider pegloticase in the tophaceous or refractory patient.

Box 2
High purine foods

- Shellfish (clams, lobster, mussels, oysters, scallops, shrimp).
- Small fish (anchovies, herring, sardines).
- Organ meats (brains, heart, kidney, liver, sweetbreads).
- Beer and overindulgence in alcohol in general.
- High fructose corn syrup enriched foods/drinks.

There is no gout diet. Reducing dietary purine burden is a small (approximately 10%) player in reducing uric acid.[8] Nevertheless the following contain fairly high amounts of purines (see **Box 2**).

CALCIUM PYROPHOSPHATE DIHYDRATE AND BASIC CALCIUM PHOSPHATE CRYSTAL DEPOSITION DISORDERS

Calcium pyrophosphate dihydrate (CPP) and basic calcium phosphate (BCP) crystals are the 2 main groups of calcium containing crystals, which can be asymptomatic or can cause painful musculoskeletal symptoms. These calcium-containing crystals can form in joints, tendons, ligaments, and soft tissue, including muscle. They are often asymptomatic and noted only as incidental findings on imaging. However, they can manifest as acute or chronic inflammatory arthritis as well as periarticular inflammatory attacks.[14]

CPP crystalline arthropathy is manifested by CPP crystal deposition in cartilage and synovial tissues. There it is called CPP deposition (CPPD). When these crystal deposits activate the immune system and cause symptoms the term CPPD disease is used. There is a marked heterogeneity of clinical presentations to this disorder. Nonetheless, as mentioned, these crystals are very often present but do not create an arthropathy. The classic radiographic finding in symptomatic or asymptomatic CPPD is punctate linear deposits of CPP crystals in the menisci or cartilage. Radiologists call this finding chondrocalcinosis. However, that is not a clinical state. Chondrocalcinosis is a common radiographic finding of CPPD deposition and does not correlate to disease manifestations very well. Symptomatic CPPD active disease is estimated at around in 1 to 5 per 1000 persons in the population[14] (**Fig. 6**).

Conditions associated with CPPD include aging, osteoarthritis, hemochromatosis, hyperparathyroidism, hypomagnesemia, and hypophosphatasia. Those metabolic derangements can be seen in the rare young patient with CPPD, as well as in the older individual. Unfortunately, correcting metabolic derangements does not seem to resolve the crystals deposited. However, correction may retard further deposition.

As with gout, the usual onset of clinical symptoms begins approximately age 55 and does not seem to have gender or ethnic/racial predilections. The overall prevalence does not seem to be increasing, as is the case with gout and hyperuricemia. Epidemiologic data are not as rich in the calcium crystal disorders as it is with hyperuricemia and gout.[14–16]

The clinical presentation of symptomatic CPPD is usually a slow onset, painful, warm monoarthritis, most often in the knee or wrist. This presentation is unlike gout, which has a very fast onset and largely affects the great toes, mid foot, or ankle in early disease. CPPD can also occur in the spine, largely at the high cervical level where it can be symptomatic.

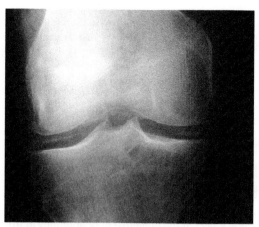

Fig. 6. CPPD radiograph of for the knee with white linear deposits in the subarticular cartilage. The menisci can be affected. This finding can be seen in other joints particularly the wrist or shoulder as well. (*Courtesy of* NL Edwards, MD.)

Despite different patterns of presentation, CPPD disease is commonly confused with gout. It is often called pseudogout for that reason. CPPD disease is a great mimicker. It can also manifest as a polyarticular noninflammatory arthritis, which is often called pseudo-osteoarthritis. Likewise, it can manifest as a polyarticular inflammatory arthritis in a pseudo-rheumatoid arthritis pattern. To complicate matters, it can present in a neuropathic-like joint destruction pattern. These terms are not useful to education a patient. More often than not, terms like "pseudo-*this*" and "pseudo-*that*" confuse the patient. Stating, "Your pain is caused by deposits of calcium crystals, not uric acid crystals. Uric acid crystals cause gout. Your condition is not gout," is a very serviceable explanation to avoid patient confusion.

When presenting as an acute or chronically inflamed joint with an effusion, a firm diagnosis rests on synovial fluid aspiration revealing rhomboid or rectangular shaped crystals with weak positive birefringence. The presence of chondrocalcinosis on plain film aid in the diagnosis. Ultrasound examination or computed tomography imagining can be useful. In usual clinic practice, these advanced modalities can often be impractical to access. As with gout, CPPD and an infected joint can overlap. Culture of synovial fluid aspirate remains the only way to rule infection out.

Unfortunately, there is no go-to therapy available to deplete calcium crystal burdens.[17] The mechanism of these ectopic calcifications remains largely unresolved. As in gout, nonsteroidal anti-inflammatory agents can moderate symptoms. Oral colchicine in the same doses used for gout is effective too. Intra-articular corticosteroids often help in the acute setting. Occasionally, in cases of persistent synovitis and repeat flares, chronic low-dose steroid therapy is needed. Making available prescriptions for burst corticosteroids steroids such as prednisone or methylprednisolone (Medrol) dose Paks to use at home for flare depends on how the disease presents.

Basic calcium crystal deposition disease (BCP) is caused by deposition of basic calcium phosphate or hydroxyapatite microcrystals mainly in extra-articular structures, such as tendons and soft tissue. Like other crystalline arthropathies, BCP crystals have a predilection for former sites of trauma. BCP deposition clinical manifestations do not typically affect more than 1 site at a time. It is often seen in patients with renal disease, diabetes, and hyperparathyroidism, as well as in aging persons, somewhat more so in older women than in older men.[17]

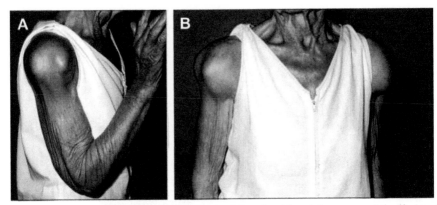

Fig. 7. Destructive arthropathy (Milwaukee) of the shoulder. A large synovial effusion is apparent over the lateral aspect of the humerus (*A*) or anteriorly in front of the glenohumeral joint (*B*). (*From* Altman RD. Clinical features of osteoarthritis. In Hochberg, M. C., Gravallese, E. M., In Silman, A. J., et al (eds). Rheumatology Elsevier: Philadelphia. 2019:1447 to 53; with permission.)

Presentations of BCP disease include a noninflammatory but destructive shoulder arthropathy largely seen in older women. This is a dramatic presentation. Called the "Milwaukee" shoulder syndrome, severe pain and loss of mobility develop rapidly and are often confused with or associated with a rotator cuff tear (**Fig. 7**). Large blood-stained joint effusions occur. The effusion can be so large, it ruptures—as a Bakers cyst in the knee can. Treatments such as aspiration or anti-inflammatory medications have variable outcomes. Total joint arthroplasty is the surgical option when conservative therapy fails.

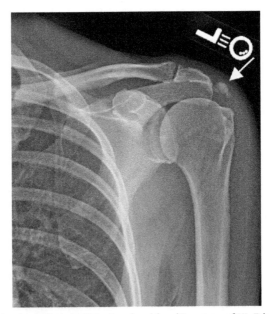

Fig. 8. Radiograph of a BCP deposit in the shoulder. (*Courtesy of* NL Edwards, MD.)

Less dramatic presentations include subacute tendonitis, often of the shoulder, wrists, or finger tendons. Acute calcific tendonitis can affect these sites. These are rarely present in more than 1 site at a time. It can be difficult to appreciate clinically if the inflammation is being generated by the joint or periarticular structure.

Laboratory features are rarely helpful other than the expected increased inflammatory markers such as the erythrocyte sedimentation rate or C-reactive protein. BCP crystals are not birefringent and cannot be seen by microscopy unless in clumps ("shiny coins"). These clumps stain with alizarin red S stain by a clinical laboratory (**Fig. 8**).

SUMMARY

Calcium-containing crystals can be associated with painful inflammatory musculoskeletal syndromes. There is not sufficient understanding of why and how these crystal deposits accrue or how they can be eliminated. In contrast with calcium-containing crystals, gout is caused by crystalline deposits of MSU. The body burden of MSU crystals can be greatly reduced, if not eliminated by urate lowering medications. Although there is no elimination therapy for excess deposits of calcium crystals, both types of crystalline arthritis can be very inflammatory and very painful. On a positive note, the suffering caused by both can be ameliorated.

Looking forward, many enthusiastic national and international research laboratories are investigating the genetic, molecular, and biochemical processes of crystalline arthropathies with steady progress toward therapies.

CLINICS CARE POINTS

- Post menopausal women can get gout.
- Don't stop allopurinol or febuxostat during a gout flare.
- Diet restrictions have modest impact on lowering uric acid. Most persons with gout require life long uric acid lowering medications.

DISCLOSURE

No disclosures.

REFERENCES

1. Kuo CF, Grainge MJ, Zhang W, et al. Global epidemiology of gout. Nat Rev Rheumatol 2015;11:649–62.
2. Cronstein BN, Sukureddi P. Mechanistic aspects of inflammation in acute gouty arthritis. J Clin Rheumatol 2015;19(1):1–29.
3. Contemporary prevalence of gout and hyperuricemia in the United States and decadal Trends: the National Health and Nutrition Examination Survey, 2007-2016. Atlanta: Center for Disease Control/National Center for Health Statistics; 2017.
4. Choi HK, Zhu Y, Mount DB, et al. The genetics of gout. Curr Opin Rheumayol 2010;22(2):144–51.
5. Roddy E, Zang W, et al. The changing epidemiology of gout. Nat Clin Pract Rheumatol 2007;3(8):443–9.
6. Keenan RT, Kransnokutsky S, JR Pillinger MH. The pathogenesis of hyperuricemia and gout. In: Firestein GS, Bubb RC, Gabriel SE, et al, editors. Kelly and

Firestone's Textbook of Rheumatology. 10th ed. Philadelphia: Elsevier Saunders; 2016. p. 1597–619.

7. Elgafy H, Liu X, Herron J. Spinal gout: a review with case illustration. World J Orthop 2016;11:766–75.

8. Terkeltaub R, Edwards NL. Gout: diagnosis and management of gouty arthritis and hyperuricemia. 4th edition. West Islip (NY): Professional Communications Inc.; 2016. p. 85–145.

9. Soltani Z, Rasheed K, Reisin E, et al. Potential role of uric acid in metabolic syndrome, hypertension, kidney injury and cardiovascular diseases. Curr Hypertens Rep 2013;15:175–81.

10. Qaseem A, Harris RP, Forciea MA, Clinical Guidelines Committee of the American College of Physicians. Management of acute and recurrent gout: a clinical practice guideline from the American College of Physicians. Ann Intern Med 2017; 166(1):58–67.

11. Khanna D, Fitzgerald JD, Khanna P, et al. 2102 American College of Rheumatology guidelines for the management of gout. Arthritis Care Res 2012;64(10): 1431–46.

12. Mikuls T. Urate-lowering therapy. In: Firestein GS, Bubb RC, Gabriel SE, et al, editors. Kelly and Firestone's Textbook of Rheumatology. 10th edition. Philadelphia: Elsevier Saunders; 2017. p. 1061–74.

13. White WB, Saag KG, Becker MA, et al. Cardiovascular safety of febuxostat or allopurinol in patients with gout. N Engl J Med 2018;378(13):1200–10.

14. Terkletaub R. Calcium crystal disease. In: Firestein GS, Bubb RC, Gabriel SE, et al, editors. Kelly and Firestone's Textbook of Rheumatology. 10th edition. Philadelphia: Elsevier Saunders; 2016. p. 1645–65.

15. Abhishek A, Doherty M. Epidemiology of calcium pyrophosphate crystal arthritis and basic calcium phosphate crystal arthropathy. Rheum Dis Clin N Am 2014;177–91.

16. Zhang W, Doherty M, Bardin T, et al. European league against rheumatism recommendations for calcium pyrophosphate deposition. Part I: terminology and diagnosis. Ann Rheum Dis 2011;70:563.

17. Weinstein E. Basic calcium phosphate and other crystalline diseases. In: West S, Kolfenbach J, editors. Rheumatology Secrets. 4th edition. Philadelphia: Elsevier Saunders; 2020. p. 380–5.

Understanding Fibromyalgia 2020

Carrie Schreibman, MSN, FNP

KEYWORDS

- Fibromyalgia • Fatigue • Nonrestorative sleep • Dyscognition

KEY POINTS

- Fibromyalgia (FM) is a disorder not only of pain but inclusive of multisystem complaints and impaired functionality.
- Diagnostic testing is not required for diagnosis. Rather, diagnosis should be based on patient report of symptoms, using a validated tool. Quantification of pain and a rating of symptom severity inclusive of fatigue, unrefreshing sleep, perceived cognitive impairment, with multisystem complaints.
- Fibromyalgia is not an autoimmune disorder, although it may exist comorbidly with other autoimmune disorders.
- Treatment goals of FM include reducing pain and symptom severity, along with maintaining functionality, improving quality of life, and preventing disability and distress.
- A multimodal treatment approach yields best outcomes: patient education, physical therapy, occupational therapy, psychotherapy, complimentary alternative medicine, and pharmacotherapy.

INTRODUCTION

Fibromyalgia (FM) is recognized as a central nervous system disorder of pain processing resulting in increased nociceptive sensitivity. It is posited that alterations in neurosensory connections result in activation of nerves that signal touch, pain, pressure, and even temperature. These changes induce amplification and distortion of sensory input. Recent research using neuroimaging demonstrates further abnormalities within brain connectivity resulting in a dysfunctional inhibitory pain network.[1] FM is characterized by chronic daily pain; overwhelming fatigue; sleep that is not refreshing; and issues with memory, word recall, and concentration. Pain is inclusive of aberrancy including but not limited to myalgia, arthralgia, neuropathic, restlessness, and spectrum sensitivities.

There is evidence suggesting neurobiologic abnormalities in FM. The hypothalamic-pituitary-adrenal axis is core to the stress adaptation response. In situations of acute stress this neuroendocrine system is adapted to protect the individual by inducing the "fight or flight" response releasing high levels of adrenal glucocorticoids. With the

Division of Arthritis and Rheumatic Diseases, Oregon Health & Science University, 3181 Southwest Sam Jackson Park Road, PV09, Portland, OR 97239, USA
E-mail address: schreibc@ohsu.edu

Physician Assist Clin 6 (2021) 89–96
https://doi.org/10.1016/j.cpha.2020.09.002
2405-7991/21/© 2020 Elsevier Inc. All rights reserved.

physicianassistant.theclinics.com

chronic prolonged stress experienced in FM, continuous exposure to cortisol and glu-cocorticoids has a paradoxic response resulting in structural and functional changes within the nervous system.[1]

HOW COMMON IS FIBROMYALGIA?

Most sources cite the prevalence of FM as anywhere from 2% to 4% with incidence being disproportionately female. FM is among the top diagnoses seen in primary care, yet it commonly takes greater than 2 years to diagnose, with an average of 3.7 consul-tation with different physicians, resulting in high medical cost and resource use.[2] The Centers for Disease Control and Prevention in 2017 estimated 4 million people are affected in the United States alone. These commonly cited statistics have been static for years and do not acknowledge increasing incidence and diversity of those affected. A literature review from 2017 estimates FM affects 0.2% to 6.6% of the gen-eral population. When divided by subcategory incidence varies dramatically: women between 2.4% and 6.8%, in urban areas between 0.7% and 11.4%, in rural areas be-tween 0.1% and 5.2%, and in special population's values between 0.6% and 15%.[3]

FM continues to be considered a woman's disorder, although there is research demonstrating FM prevalence is similar among males and females.[4] Depending on the diagnostic criteria applied, prevalence of the disorder in males varies.[5] Historical use of the 1990 criteria, requiring clinician input, possibly subject to bias, using the ten-der point examination, underestimates the number of males affected and may skew male to female incidence. Use of the modified 2010 criteria, patient report with use of a validated tool is objective and has contributed to increased diagnosis among males.[5,6]

WHAT ARE THE DIAGNOSTIC DILEMMAS?

There is presently no gold standard for diagnosis. There are multiple criteria for diag-nosis in use currently. The most commonly used criteria, 1990 and 2010, are delin-eated here.

Classification Criteria

Not since the American College of Rheumatology 1990 Criteria for Diagnosis[7] has there been consensus. The 1990 criteria assess "tender points" throughout the body, with 4 kg of pressure applied to each point. There are 18 qualified points with diagnosis being positive for 11 or more points in the context of pain greater than 3-month duration and not of other known cause.[8] The 1990 criteria have a myriad of limitations. It is impractical for use in the clinical setting, in that there is a lack of con-fidence among nonrheumatology providers confused by specificity of points and application of pressure.[9] It is reductionist, in that the sole focus on pain does not include commonly associated symptoms or severity of pain.[8]

The 2010 preliminary criteria[10] ushered in recognition of FM as a multisystem disor-der inclusive of widespread chronic pain, fatigue, dyscognition, and nonrestorative sleep.[10] Critics contend this approach draws away from chronic pain as the core symptom of the disorder.

The 2010 Preliminary Diagnostic Criteria for Fibromyalgia simplifies diagnosis for nonrheumatology providers with quantification of two scales. Diagnostic criteria are met if the patient has a Widespread Pain Index of seven or more with a Symptom Severity Score of five or more or a Widespread Pain Index of three to six with a Symp-tom Severity Score of nine or more (**Box 1, Tables 1–3**). These scores are in the context of consistent symptoms for 3 or more months and no other disorder that would explain the pain.

> **Box 1**
> **American College of Rheumatology 2010 diagnostic criteria for fibromyalgia**
>
> Must meet all three conditions:
> 1. Widespread Pain Index ≥7 plus Symptom Severity Score ≥5 or Widespread Pain Index 3 to 6 plus Symptom Severity Score ≥9.
> 2. Symptoms have been present for 3 or more months.
> 3. The patient does not have another disorder that would explain the pain.
>
> *Data from* Manga Wolfe F, Clauw DJ, Fitzcharles MA, et al. The American College of Rheumatology preliminary diagnostic criteria for fibromyalgia and measurement of symptom severity. *Arthritis Care Res.* 2010; 62(5): 600-610.

FACTORS COMPLICATING DIAGNOSIS

Patients with FM tend to have multiple comorbidities including chronic low back pain, irritable bowel syndrome, dysautonomia, osteoarthritis, migraine, chronic daily headache, interstitial cystitis, dysmenorrhea, mood disorders, and post-traumatic stress disorder. Clinicians may feel overwhelmed by these complaints and focus on one or two without developing a global clinical impression. In patients, cognitive dissonance is a common response to diagnosis. Psychological distress and questioning of accurate diagnosis is common.[11]

There also may be confusion if the tender point examination is used. The tender points identified overlap with sites of enthesitis found in spondyloarthritis.[12] There are several ongoing studies looking at the incidence of FM in spondyloarthritis.

Furthermore, there is misconception that FM is an autoimmune disease. There is no basis for autoimmunity in FM, although 30% of patients with other rheumatologic disease do comorbidly have FM. It is a central nervous system (neurosensory) disorder with neuroendocrine features.

CLINICAL FEATURES
Pain

In FM there is widespread, generalized pain that is chronic in origin. Allodynia, pain experienced from a nonnoxious stimulus, such as sensitivity to touch, can be pathognomonic. Hyperalgesia, abnormally heightened sensitivity to pain, is an additional core finding.

Table 1
Widespread Pain Index: patient report of pain in the following locations in the last week

Right	Left	
Shoulder girdle	Shoulder girdle	Neck
Upper arm	Upper arm	Upper back
Lower arm	Lower arm	Lower back
Hip (buttock or trochanter)	Hip (buttock or trochanter)	Chest
Upper leg	Upper leg	Abdomen
Lower leg	Lower leg	Head
Jaw	Jaw	Total

Score 0 to 19.

Data from Wolfe F, Clauw DJ, Fitzcharles MA, et al. The American College of Rheumatology preliminary diagnostic criteria for fibromyalgia and measurement of symptom severity. *Arthritis Care Res.* 2010; 62(5): 600-610.

Table 2
Symptom Severity Score (part 1): indicate the level of symptom severity over the past week

Fatigue	Sleep	Cognitive
0 = no problems	0 = no problems	0 = no problems
1 = mild or intermittent problem	1 = mild or intermittent problem	1 = mild or intermittent problem
2 = moderate problem	2 = moderate problem	2 = moderate problem
3 = severe, pervasive, life altering	3 = severe, pervasive, life altering	3 = severe, pervasive, life altering
Total	Total	Total

Score 0 to 9.
   Data from Wolfe F, Clauw DJ, Fitzcharles MA, et al. The American College of Rheumatology preliminary diagnostic criteria for fibromyalgia and measurement of symptom severity. *Arthritis Care Res.* 2010; 62(5): 600-610.

Fatigue

Fatigue is central to the diagnosis. Chronic fatigue syndrome is not consistent with FM and the terms should not be used interchangeably.

Sleep Disturbance

In FM there is nonrestorative sleep as evidenced by waking feeling unrefreshed. The pathophysiology of impaired restful sleep stems from intrusion of alpha wave sleep on delta wave. Myriad sleep disorders may coexist with FM including insomnia, restless leg syndrome, sleep apnea, and upper airway resistance syndrome.

Dyscognition

Most patients complain of cognitive concerns. Issues with short-term memory, word recall, linear thinking, focus, and problem solving are commonly reported. This is commonly referred to as "fibro fog."

LABORATORY TESTING

Diagnostic testing is not necessary to make the diagnosis of FM. However, evaluating for common comorbid disorders may be helpful.

1. Erythrocyte sedimentation rate: Although sensitive, it is not specific. Erythrocyte sedimentation rate is a useful tool in differentiating an inflammatory versus noninflammatory disorder if there is concern.

Table 3
Symptom Severity Score (part 2): indicate the number of positive reports of review of symptoms in the last week

0	= 0
1–10	= 1
11–24	= 2
25 or more	= 3

Add score 0 to 3 to score from part 1 to determine the total symptom severity index.
   Data from Wolfe F, Clauw DJ, Fitzcharles MA, et al. The American College of Rheumatology preliminary diagnostic criteria for fibromyalgia and measurement of symptom severity. *Arthritis Care Res.* 2010; 62(5): 600-610.

2. Vitamin D 25-OH: Hypovitaminosis D is linked to increased arthralgia, myalgia, fatigue, and circadian rhythm disturbance. Repletion and maintenance of adequate levels of vitamin D may minimize these symptoms.[13]
3. Thyroid-stimulating hormone: Thyroid disorders, particularly hypothyroid, may be a cofactor contributing to worsening fatigue and/or depression. Ensuring hypothyroid is not present as a new diagnosis or confirming adequate treatment of known disease by normal thyroid-stimulating hormone is helpful.
4. Complete blood count with differential: Screening for anemia or other blood dyscrasias that may be contributory to and/or identify other disorders beyond FM.
5. Hepatitis C virus antibody: Hepatitis C is often an invisible disease. Musculoskeletal complaints and fatigue are common in hepatitis C virus as they are in FM. Comorbid hepatitis C virus complicates the FM clinical picture. Because treatment is now available, testing for hepatitis C virus is encouraged.
6. Insulin-like growth factor 1: Patients with FM tend to have lower levels of growth hormone. Some may have growth hormone deficiency. Growth hormone deficiency symptoms include fatigue, myalgia, and depression. If present comorbidly, treatment could improve these core symptoms.

IMAGING

No imaging is necessary to substantiate diagnosis.

MANAGEMENT
Patient Education

Patient education is the single most important intervention. Often these patients have struggled with their symptoms for years without tangible diagnosis. It is common that they have been referred to multiple specialists and completed extensive laboratory and imaging studies to no avail. FM affects every aspect of the patient's life and fear of serious, yet treatable illness is paramount to them.

Physical Therapy and Exercise

The European League Against Rheumatism 2016 guidelines for the treatment of FM give exercise therapy their highest recommendation.[14] Often patients with FM are deconditioned and need expert assistance and direction to safely develop an effective exercise program. Aerobic and muscle strengthening exercises are recommended. Exercise is the most effective way to improve pain and depression in patients with FM. Stretching with aerobic activity has been shown to increase health-related quality of life measures.[15]

Occupational Therapy

Occupational therapy is a discipline commonly overlooked when dealing with chronic pain and functional disorders in the outpatient setting. Occupational therapy has validated practice guidelines for adults with arthritis and other rheumatic conditions, such as FM.[16] Occupational therapy focuses on energy-conservation strategies, leading to increased endurance and strength remediation, which are extremely helpful for patients with FM dealing with fatigue.[16]

Pain Psychology

Although there is a high comorbid incidence of mental health disorders, pain itself leads to or perpetuates depression, anxiety, and panic. Use of standard cognitive behavioral therapy is recommended for patients with depression and anxiety.

Acceptance and commitment therapy have proven benefit for all individuals living with chronic pain. Acceptance and commitment therapy encourages self-acceptance through mindfulness. Research demonstrates that acceptance and commitment therapy has greatest impact on pain-related functioning and mental health–related quality of life measures.[17]

Complementary Alternative Medicine

Because of few affective therapies for dealing with pain in FM, many patients turn to varied forms of complementary alternative medicine. There are only three complementary alternative medicines with data to support use ranging from moderate to weak: (1) pain psychology, (2) acupuncture, and (3) chiropractic and massage.[18]

Pharmacotherapy

Efficacy of pharmacotherapies is limited because there are no specific pathophysiologic therapeutic targets for treatment.[13] Many commonly used medications in the treatment of FM, FDA approved and off-label, are serotonergic in nature. Polypharmacy is often seen in these patients with duplication of serotonergic agents commonly found. This poses risk for a spectrum of serotoninergic toxicity.[19]

Food and Drug Administration–approved drugs approved for treatment of fibromyalgia

1. Selective serotonin norepinephrine reuptake inhibitors (SNRIs) increase levels of inhibitory neurotransmitters. Duloxetine is an SNRI, Food and Drug Administration (FDA) approved in the treatment of FM. Maximum effective dosing is 60 mg daily. Duloxetine has a myriad of other indications including major depressive disorder. It is an agent that works best in patients with comorbid depression. Milnacipran is another SNRI approved for treatment of FM. Therapeutic dosing is 50 to 100 mg twice daily. Milnacipran came late to the US market and is only indicated for FM. These factors may be contributory to its less common use.
2. Pregabalin is an anticonvulsant FDA approved for treatment of FM. Anticonvulsants decrease levels of excitatory neurotransmitters. It is structurally like the neurotransmitter γ-aminobutyric acid but does not have activity within the γ-aminobutyric acid neuronal system. The analgesic effect is exerted by binding voltage-fated calcium channels in the central nervous system. Therapeutic dosing is 150 mg twice to three times daily.[14]

Drugs commonly used off-label in fibromyalgia

1. Gabapentin functions similarly to pregabalin, although it is not FDA approved for treating FM. It is commonly used off-label in many chronic pain conditions including FM. Therapeutic dosing is unknown for FM.[14]
2. Amitriptyline is a tricyclic antidepressant that inhibits serotonin and noradrenaline reuptake. It is most used off-label in the treatment of neuropathic pain and FM. Limited studies have found benefit with use between 10 and 50 mg/d.[14]
3. Cyclobenzaprine is a skeletal muscle relaxant. European League Against Rheumatism 2017 endorses use off-label in moderate to severe FM particularly in those with sleep disturbance. Initial dosing is endorsed as 5 to 10 mg before bed. Titration is up to 40 mg in one to three doses daily as needed and tolerated.
4. Tramadol is classified as an opiate analgesic. Use of conventional opiates in FM is generally not recommended. Pharmacologically tramadol is different; it is a synthetic opioid receptor antagonist with dominant SNRI properties.[20] Research has demonstrated benefit in FM as a second-line treatment of more severe cases.[18]

Emerging Therapies

Cannabinoids
Dysregulation of the endocannabinoid system in pain modulation and in FM is hypothesized. Cannabinoids are being investigated in treating chronic pain. There are two major active compounds in cannabinoids: tetrahydrocannabinol and cannabidiol. Tetrahydrocannabinol has psychoactive properties that have effect on pain and mood via the CB1 and CB2 receptors. CB1 receptors are within the central nervous system and peripheral nervous system and act as agonists along sensory pathways as modulators of pain. Selective CB1 agonists, with little to no presence of tetrahydrocannabinol, are being investigated for use.[21]

N-methyl-ᴅ-aspartate antagonists
Glutamate is the most abundant excitatory neurotransmitter in the nervous system. Central sensitization is associated with hyperexcitability of the glutaminergic system. N-methyl-ᴅ-aspartate is one of three groups of glutamate receptors. High levels of glutamate have been identified in the brains of patients with FM. Antagonizing the N-methyl-ᴅ-aspartate receptor to reduce glutamate levels theoretically should decrease the severity of FM pain.[20]

SUMMARY AND DISCUSSION

FM is a chronic functional illness of widespread pain, fatigue, nonrestorative sleep, and cognitive complaints. Allodynia and hyperalgesia are hallmark features of the disorder. Prevalence of FM is most commonly estimated to be 2% to 4% of the population with approximately 4 million people in the United States affected. Currently there is no one criteria for diagnosis beyond the 1990 tender point examination. The tender point examination is difficult for most clinicians to perform and/or interpret and may be subject to bias. The proposed 2010 and subsequent criteria propose an objective patient self-report of symptoms validated using a standardized tool in light of a normal examination and no other reason for symptoms. FM has been thought to be a disorder of women. Using the 2010 criteria male to female incidence is increasing. A multimodal approach to care is recommended.

CLINICS CARE POINTS

- Primary care providers diagnose and treat fibromyalgia.
- Patient education at diagnosis is critical: Etiology, implications, treatment, monitoring and prognosis.
- Multi-modality treatment approaches provide the best outcomes.
- Many of the pharmacologic agents used to treat fibromyalgia are serotonergic.
- Polypharmacy is common in fibromyalgia patients and places them at risk for the spectrum of serotonergic toxicity which can mimic worsening fibromyalgia symptoms.
- Effectively treat comorbid conditions which may be present.

REFERENCES

1. Pamfil C, Choy EHS. Functional MRI in rheumatic diseases with a focus on fibromyalgia. Clin Exp Rheumatol 2018;36 Suppl 114(5):82–5.

2. Macfarlane GJ, Kronisch C, Dean LE, et al. EULAR revised recommendations for the management of fibromyalgia. Ann Rheum Dis 2017;76(2):318–28.

3. Marques AP, Santo ASDE, Berssaneti AA, et al. Prevalence of fibromyalgia: literature review update. Rev Bras Reumatol Engl Ed 2017;57(4):356–63.
4. Muraleetharan D, Fadich A, Stephenson C, et al. Understanding the impact of fibromyalgia on men: findings from a nationwide survey. Am J Mens Health 2018; 12(4):952–60.
5. Heidari F, Afshari M, Moosazadeh M. Prevalence of fibromyalgia in general population and patients, a systematic review and meta-analysis. Rheumatol Int 2017; 37(9):1527–39.
6. Häuser W, Fitzcharles MA. Facts and myths pertaining to fibromyalgia. Dialogues Clin Neurosci 2018;20(1):53–62.
7. Wolfe F, Smythe HA, Yunus MB, et al. The American College of Rheumatology 1990 criteria for the classification of fibromyalgia: report of the Multicenter Criteria Committee. Arthritis Rheum 1990;33:160–72.
8. Harden RN, Revivo G, Song S, et al. A critical analysis of the tender points in fibromyalgia. Pain Med 2007;8(2):147–56.
9. Arnold LM, Bennett RM, Crofford LJ, et al. AAPT diagnostic criteria for fibromyalgia. J Pain 2019;20:611–28.
10. Wolfe F, Clauw DJ, Fitzcharles MA, et al. The American College of Rheumatology preliminary diagnostic criteria for fibromyalgia and measurement of symptom severity. Arthritis Care Res 2010;62(5):600-610.
11. Gendelman O, Amital H, Bar-On Y, et al. Time to diagnosis of fibromyalgia and factors associated with delayed diagnosis in primary care. Best Pract Res Clin Rheumatol 2018;32(4):489–99.
12. Roussou E, Ciurtin C. Clinical overlap between fibromyalgia tender points and enthesitis sites in patients with spondyloarthritis who present with inflammatory back pain. Clin Exp Rheumatol 2012;30(6 Suppl 74):24–30.
13. Martins YA, Cardinali CAEF, Ravanelli MI, et al. Is hypovitaminosis D associated with fibromyalgia? A systematic review. Nutr Rev 2020;78(2):115–33.
14. Kia S, Choy E. Update on treatment guideline in fibromyalgia syndrome with focus on pharmacology. Biomedicine 2017;5(2):20.
15. Sosa-Reina MD, Nunez-Nagy S, Gallego-Izquierdo T, et al. Effectiveness of therapeutic exercise in fibromyalgia syndrome: a systematic review and meta-analysis of randomized clinical trials. Biomed Res Int 2017;2017:2356346.
16. Siegel P, Jones BL, Poole JL. Occupational therapy interventions for adults with fibromyalgia. Am J Occup Ther 2018;72(5). 7205395010p1–7205395010p4.
17. Wicksell RK, Kemani M, Jensen K, et al. Acceptance and commitment therapy for fibromyalgia: a randomized controlled trial. Eur J Pain 2013;17(4):599–611.
18. Berman BM, Swyers JP. Complementary medicine treatments for fibromyalgia syndrome. Baillieres Best Pract Res Clin Rheumatol 1999;13(3):487–92.
19. Isbister GK, Buckley NA, Whyte IM. Serotonin toxicity: a practical approach to diagnosis and treatment. Med J Aust 2007;187(6):361–5.
20. MacLean AJ, Schwartz TL. Tramadol for the treatment of fibromyalgia. Expert Rev Neurother 2015;15(5):469–75.
21. Tzadok R, Ablin JN. Current and emerging pharmacotherapy for fibromyalgia. Pain Res Manag 2020;2020:6541798.

Idiopathic Inflammatory Myositis

Michael G. Feely, MD

KEYWORDS

- Myositis • Idiopathic inflammatory myopathies • Dermatomyositis • Polymyositis
- Anti-synthetase syndrome • Inclusion body myositis

KEY POINTS

- Idiopathic inflammatory myopathies (IIMs) are systemic autoimmune disorders character-ized by muscular inflammation, leading to proximal muscle weakness and poor muscular endurance.
- Extramuscular manifestations are common and may affect the skin, lungs, gastrointestinal tract, and heart.
- Myositis-specific antibodies aid in the classification of patients and correlate with specific clinical phenotypes.
- Corticosteroids and immunosuppressive medications are the mainstay of treatment, although exercise recently has been shown to be an integral part of the management of IIMs.

INTRODUCTION

Idiopathic inflammatory myopathies (IIMs) are a group of heterogenous systemic auto-immune disorders, collectively termed, *myositis*, characterized by muscle weakness and poor muscular endurance and often accompanied by extramuscular manifesta-tions involving the skin, lungs, gastrointestinal tract, and joints. Classically, IIMs were categorized as dermatomyositis (DM), polymyositis (PM), or inclusion body myositis (IBM), but amyopathic forms and immune-mediated necrotizing myopathies (IMNMs) now are recognized. Identification of myositis-specific antibodies (MSAs) has contributed to the classification of IIMs and are associated with distinct clinical phe-notypes and often are of prognostic value. IIMs are rare disorders, with an incidence of 11 per million, and affect both adult and pediatric populations.[1] Given the multisys-temic involvement of IIMs and the potential for the extramuscular manifestations to be the initial symptoms, patients may present to primary care physicians, physicians

Department of Internal Medicine, Division of Rheumatology, University of Nebraska Medical Center, 986270 Nebraska Medical Center, Omaha, NE 68198-6270, USA
E-mail address: mfeely@unmc.edu

Physician Assist Clin 6 (2021) 97–109
https://doi.org/10.1016/j.cpha.2020.08.006
2405-7991/21/© 2020 Elsevier Inc. All rights reserved.

assistants, nurse practitioners, rheumatologists, dermatologists, pulmonologists, or neurologists.

CLINICAL CHARACTERISTICS

Although the different IIMs often present similarly, they have epidemiologic, serologic, and histologic differences. Furthermore, prognosis, treatment strategies, and potential for extramuscular manifestations differ among the subtypes. IIMs typically present with the insidious onset of symmetric proximal muscle weakness, although IBM also often involves distal muscles and may have an asymmetric distribution. Patients may experience difficulties performing tasks requiring the use of the proximal musculature, such as climbing stairs, rising from a seated position, and washing their hair. Given the distal involvement in IBM, patients may have difficulty with tasks, such as buttoning shirts, writing, and manipulating coins. The neck flexors and pharyngeal musculature frequently are involved in IIMs and may lead to head drop and dysphagia, respectively. In advanced cases, the respiratory muscles can be affected. Ocular muscles are spared in all IIMs, and, although the facial muscles are not affected in DM/PM, they can be involved in IBM. DM has a female predilection, with a bimodal age of onset of 5 years to 15 years and 45 years to 65 years. PM rarely occurs in children. IBM typically occurs after age 50 and disproportionately affects males moreso than female.

DERMATOMYOSITIS

Several characteristic rashes are seen in DM. Gottron papules are erythematous, papular lesions occurring over the interphalangeal joints of the hands (**Fig. 1**) and extensor surfaces of elbows and knees. The heliotrope rash is a violaceous rash of the eyelids and often accompanied by periorbital edema. Both the heliotrope rash and Gottron papules are specific for DM. Other rashes, including the V sign (erythema of the anterior aspect of neck), shawl sign (erythema of upper back), periungual erythema, and holster sign (erythema of lateral aspect of thighs), are common, although not specific for DM. The cutaneous lesions of DM often worsen with exposure to ultraviolet light and can be quite pruritic.

Amyopathic forms of DM occur and are characterized by the classic rashes of DM but also may have extramuscular features, such as interstitial lung disease (ILD), dysphagia,

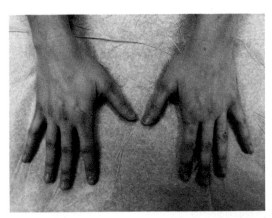

Fig. 1. Gottron papules on a patient with DM; note the periungual erythema often seen in DM.

and malignancy. Some patients ultimately develop muscle weakness, whereas others remain amyopathic. Amyopathic DM associated with antibodies to melanoma differentiation-associated gene 5 (MDA-5) has a unique clinical phenotype characterized by classic lesions of DM as well as ulcerative and papular lesions and in some populations has been associated with development of rapidly progressive ILD.[2–4]

Juvenile DM (JDM) is a rare disorder, with an incidence of 2 million to 4 per million, with an increased risk in females.[5] A majority of patients with JDM are autoantibody positive, with antibodies to nucleosome-modifying deacetylase complex (Mi-2), nuclear matrix protein 2 (NXP-2), transcription intermediary factor 1 gamma (TIF1-γ), and MDA-5 the most common. JDM patients may have profound muscle weakness and prominent skin rashes. Calcinosis is a much more frequent complication of JDM than in adult DM and can be associated with significant morbidity. Some patients can have a prominent vasculopathy. Antisynthetase syndrome and amyopathic variants are rare in children.

POLYMYOSITIS

Due to shifts in approach to classification of IIMs, namely increased recognition of IMNMs as a distinct subtype, PM has become a rare diagnosis. Because of overlapping symptoms and histopathologic similarities, IBM, IMNMs, and muscular dystrophies often are misdiagnosed as PM. PM now is considered a diagnosis of exclusion. It presents with proximal muscle weakness, similar to DM, although skin rashes are absent. It occurs almost exclusively in adults and can coexist with other connective tissue disorders, including systemic sclerosis, systemic lupus erythematosus (SLE), and mixed connective tissue disease. Given the clinical similarities between IBM and PM, it is imperative to exclude IBM by muscle biopsy, given the differing prognoses and approach to treatment.

ANTISYNTHETASE SYNDROME

Antisynthetase syndrome is a subset of IIMs characterized by the presence of myositis, fever, raynaud's phenomenon, a non-erosive inflammatory arthritis, mechanic's hands—prominent dry, fissured skin on fingers (**Fig. 2**), and ILD, occurring in patients with antibodies to transfer RNA (tRNA) synthetases—enzymes that play and important role in protein synthesis. Eight synthetase antibodies have been described, although the most common of these are antibodies targeting the histidyl-

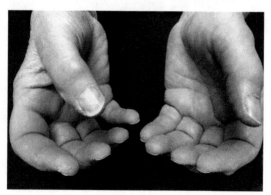

Fig. 2. Mechanic's hands in a patient with Jo-1[+] antisynthetase syndrome.

tRNA synthetase (Jo-1).[6] Patients with antisynthetase syndrome may fulfill criteria for either DM or PM. Patients with antisynthetase syndrome are at high risk for developing ILD (**Fig. 3**).

IMMUNE-MEDIATED NECROTIZING MYOPATHIES

IMNMs present similarly to DM/PM, although often are characterized by greater elevations of muscle enzymes, and myalgias are more common than in other IIMs. Patients may have severe weakness at presentation. Histologically, prominent necrosis of the myofibril occurs with scant inflammatory cell infiltrates. Antibodies to the signal recognition particle (SRP) and hydroxy-methyl guanosine coenzyme A reductase (HMGCR) are associated with IMNMs. Exposure to statin medications, which inhibit cholesterol synthesis by targeting the HMGCR enzyme, occasionally results in the development of antibodies to HMGCR and a necrotizing myopathy. Unlike other myotoxic effects of statins, discontinuation of these agents alone is not sufficient, because immunosuppressive or immunomodulatory therapies also are needed. Necrotizing histologies can be seen in JDM, occasionally with the presence of SRP or HMGCR antibodies (even in statin-naïve patients).

INCLUSION BODY MYOSITIS

IBM is the most common acquired myopathy, occurring after 50 years of age, and has a male predilection. It presents with weakness and atrophy of the distal musculature, in particular the foot extensors and deep finger flexors. Involvement of the quadriceps and forearms occurs early in the disease and often leads to prominent atrophy. Falls are common due to the quadriceps weakness and resultant instability. Dysphagia is common, occurring in approximately 50% of patients, and results in an increased risk for aspiration pneumonias.[7] IBM tends to progress slowly and is associated with significant disability, with most patients ultimately requiring assistive devices, such as canes, walkers, and wheelchairs, within 10 years of diagnosis. IBM is not associated with an increased risk for ILD, cutaneous lesions, malignancies, or arthritis.

DIAGNOSTIC EVALUATION

The evaluation of a patient with suspected myosites depends on the presenting features. Given the heterogeneity of these disorders, patients may present with

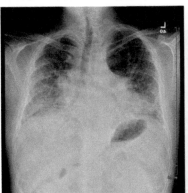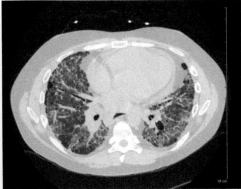

Fig. 3. Chest radiograph and corresponding computed tomography scan of patient with ILD associated with Jo-1⁺ antisynthetase syndrome.

complaints of skin rashes, muscle weakness, or shortness of breath. When evaluating a weak patient, it is imperative to determine whether the patient has true muscle weakness, because myalgia often can lead to the perception of weakness. The differential diagnosis of muscle weakness is broad and includes endocrinopathies, metabolic disorders, and neurologic disease, among several other etiologies of weakness (**Box 1**). Measurement of muscle enzymes, including creatine kinase (CK), aldolase, lactate dehydrogenase, aspartate transaminase, and alanine transaminase, often is among the first tests done to evaluate a patient with muscle weakness. Although muscle enzymes typically are elevated, these abnormalities are not specific for IIMs, and, by contrast, normal muscle enzymes do not exclude IIMs. Serum levels of CK may be elevated to 50 times the upper limit of normal in IMNMs and DM, although typically are less elevated in IBM (up to 10 times the upper limit of normal). The diagnostic work-up also should evaluate for other causes of muscle weakness, including endocrinopathies, electrolyte abnormalities, and other systemic illness.

Box 1
Differential diagnosis of idiopathic inflammatory myopathies

Endocrinopathies
- Hypothyroidism
- Hyperthyroidism
- Acromegaly
- Cushing syndrome
- Adrenal insufficiency

Toxins/medications
- Statins
- Ethanol
- Colchicine
- Antipsychotics
- Hydroxychloroquine
- Cocaine/amphetamines
- L-Tryptophan

Neuromuscular disorders
- Muscular dystrophies
- Myasthenia gravis
- Eaton-Lambert syndrome
- Denervating syndromes
- Guillain-Barré syndrome
- Amyotrophic lateral sclerosis

Infections
- Bacterial
- Viral (human immunodeficiency virus, influenza, coxsackie, hepatitis B)
- Parasitic (toxoplasmosis, trichinellosis, schistosomiasis, cysticercosis)

Metabolic
- Glycogen storage diseases
- Carnitine deficiency/carnitine palmitoyl transferase deficiency
- Mitochondrial myopathies
- Vitamin deficiencies (vitamin D, vitamin E)
- Electrolyte deficiencies (hypokalemia, hypocalcemia, hypercalcemia, hyperphosphatemia)

Others
- Amyloidosis
- Rhabdomyolysis
- Sarcoidosis

Electromyography (EMG) often is helpful in evaluating weakness and can differentiate between myopathic and neurogenic etiologies. Characteristic findings on EMG of a patient with an active inflammatory myopathy include myopathic motor unit potentials characterized by short-duration, low-amplitude polyphasic units; fibrillations; complex repetitive discharges; and positive sharp waves. Although not diagnostic of an IIM, these EMG findings are supportive and may help with identification of an appropriate site for biopsy. EMG cannot differentiate IIMs from toxic myopathies or dystrophies. Magnetic resonance imaging (MRI) increasingly is utilized in the evaluation for IIMs. Short tau inversion recovery and fat-suppressed T2 sequences on MRI can identify muscle edema suggesting active inflammation, and T1 sequences may reveal fatty replacement of muscle and scar tissue, suggesting long-standing or aggressive disease. In addition to evaluating for inflammatory changes, MRI can be useful in identifying a site for biopsy and assessing disease activity.[8]

Despite advances in imaging and serologic studies, muscle biopsy remains the gold standard for diagnosis (**Table 1**). Histologic analysis of muscle biopsies in DM is demonstrate perivascular T-cell and B-cell infiltrates, with non-necrotic muscle fibers and membrane attack complex deposition in the vessel walls. PM is characterized histologically by an endomysial infiltrate composed of $CD8^+$ T cells and increased expression of major histocompatibility complex (MHC) class I. IMNMs are characterized by abundant necrosis with scant cellular infiltrates, although MHC class I also is up-regulated. IBM can show features similar to those in PM, including $CD8^+$ T-cell infiltrate and up-regulation of MHC class I but has chronic myopathic changes and autophagic vacuoles and tubulofilamentous inclusions. Up to 30% of patients with an IBM phenotype, however, do not show vacuoles or inclusions on biopsy.[9] In patients with classic rashes of DM and a consistent clinical picture, a muscle biopsy may not be necessary. In patients presenting with suspected amyopathic DM, a skin biopsy can be helpful to rule out other mimics.

Table 1
Characteristics of idiopathic inflammatory myopathy subtypes

Idiopathic Inflammatory Myopathy	Epidemiology	Clinical	Histopathology
DM	Female > male Ages 5–15 and 45–65	Proximal weakness Rashes, calcinosis, ulcerations ILD Increased malignancy	Perivascular inflammation, perifascicular atrophy
PM	Adults	Proximal weakness No rashes ILD	Endomysial inflammation, $CD8^+$ T-cells, up-regulated MHC-1 expression
IMNM	Most common in adults, though occasionally in children Often with SRP or HMGCR antibodies	Proximal muscle weakness. CK up to 50× upper limits of normal Myalgia common	Prominent necrosis, scant inflammation
IBM	Age >50 y Male > female	Proximal and distal weakness. Dysphagia common No proved treatments	Endomysial inflammation, tubulofilamentous inclusion, rimmed vacuoles

MYOSITIS ANTIBODIES

Autoimmunity is known to play a role in the pathogenesis of IIMs, and autoantibodies are present in more than half of patients with IIMs. Several MSAs and myositis-associated antibodies (MAAs) have been identified and have both prognostic and diagnostic value (**Table 2**). Additionally, these biomarkers have contributed to the classification of IIMs and can correlate with specific phenotypes. MSAs, as their name suggests, have high specificity for IIMs, and generally are mutually exclusive. MAAs are not specific for IIMs and often are seen in other connective tissue disorders or in myositis overlap syndromes.

Antisynthetase antibodies are a group of antibodies directed against tRNA synthetases and are associated with the clinical features of antisynthetase syndrome. Antibodies to tRNA synthetases are seen in 25% to 35% of patients with IIMs.[10] The most common of the 8 antisynthetase antibodies is Jo-1, which targets histidyl-tRNA synthetase, occurring in 9% to 24% of adult IIMs.[6] Although the clinical phenotype of antisynthetase syndrome has similarities among these various antibodies, there are clinical differences as well, particularly with respect to the frequency and presence of rashes and the timing of myositis onset.[11] Prognosis of IIMs differs among

Table 2 Myositis antibodies	

Antisynthetase antibodies
  Jo-1
  PL-7
  PL-12
  KS
  OJ
  Zo
  EJ
  Ha
	Antisynthetase syndrome
	• Inflammatory arthritis
	• Fever
	• Myositis
	• ILD
	• Raynaud phenomenon
	• Mechanic's hands

Mi-2	DM; rashes, myositis, good response to treatment
SAE	DM; rash, myositis
MDA-5	Amyopathic DM, rash, ulcers, palmar papules, rapidly progressive ILD
NXP-2	DM; prominent rash, calcinosis in kids, associated with malignancy in adults
TIF1-γ	DM; rash, strong association with malignancy in adults
SRP	IMNM; often severe myopathy
HMGCR	IMNM: statin associated (in most cases)
5NT1a	IBM
Ku	Overlap myositis
SnRNP	Overlap myositis
Ro	CTD related myositis
La	CTD related myositis
PM/Scl	Scleroderma/myositis overlap

Abbreviation: DM, dermatomyositis.

different antibody groups, because antisynthetase syndrome patients with antibodies to Jo-1 have better 5-year and 10-year survival rates compared with those who have non–Jo-1 antibodies.[12]

Several other MSAs that associate with DM have been described. Antibodies to small ubiquitin-like modifier activating enzyme (SAE) and Mi-2 are characterized by classic skin lesions and muscle weakness but are not associated with an increased risk of ILD. Although muscle weakness can be profound, the presence of Mi-2 antibodies correlates with a favorable response to treatment. Antibodies to TIF1-γ are associated with severe skin involvement and more importantly associate with an increased risk of malignancy.[13] Antibodies to NXP-2 are seen in both JDM and adult DM. In JDM, these antibodies correlate with the presence of calcinosis, whereas in adult DM, they associate with an increased risk of malignancy.[14] Antibodies to melanoma differentiation gene 5 (MDA-5) are associated with amyopathic DM with severe skin involvement, including typical DM lesions but also cutaneous ulcers, panniculitis, palmar papules, and an increased risk for rapidly progressing ILD (particularly in Asian cohorts).[2]

Both antibodies to hydroxyl-methyl guanosine coenzyme A reductase (HMGCR) and SRP are associated with necrotizing forms of IIMs. Antibodies to HMGCR typically are seen in patients treated with statins, although this antibody has been identified in statin-naïve IIM patients as well.[15] Antibodies to SRP are seen in 5% to 10% patients with IIMs and are associated with a severe myopathy with rapidly progressive weakness often refractory to therapy.

IBM typically is considered a degenerative myopathy with secondary inflammation. Although autoantibodies are not classically associated with IBM, a small portion of patients are autoantibody positive. Antibodies to cytosolic 5′ nucleotidase 1a have been identified in 33% to 34% of patients with IBM.[16,17] These antibodies are not specific for IBM and have been identified in other connective tissue disorders, including Sjögren syndrome and SLE.

FURTHER EVALUATION

Once a diagnosis of myositis is established, it is necessary to evaluate for extramuscular manifestations. A thorough history and physical examination may identify symptoms of extramuscular involvement guide further studies. Given the association of ILD with IIMs, chest radiography, high-resolution computed tomography of the chest, and pulmonary function testing often are indicated. The presence of specific MSAs may help guide these investigations. Myocardial involvement of IIMs rarely is of clinical significance but can be associated with high mortality and morbidity; thus, it is necessary to maintain a high index of suspicion for cardiac involvement, and electrocardiograms and echocardiography may be warranted. Dysphagia may complicate IIMs, particularly in IBM, requiring evaluation with video esophagrams and speech therapy.

The association of IIMs and malignancy has long been recognized. This is true particularly for DM, which is characterized by an up to 8-fold increase in the risk of cancer in the 3 years prior to and after the diagnosis of DM.[14,18,19] The spectrum of malignancies associated with DM typically resembles that of the general population. PM and IMNMs are characterized by an increased risk of malignancy relative to the general population, albeit to a much lesser extent than seen in DM. IBM is not characterized by an increased risk of malignancy. MSAs can be instructive regarding the risk for malignancy, because the presence of antibodies to TIF1-γ and NXP-2 (in adults) is strongly associated with malignancy.[13] Screening for malignancy is imperative at the time of diagnosis of an IIM, in particular DM. There are no specific recommendations regarding the screening approach, although it generally is well agreed on that it should be ensured that age-appropriate screening is performed, and often CT of the chest, abdomen, and pelvis is performed as well as a gynecologic ultrasound in women. For particularly high-risk patients, PET may be warranted.[14] The frequency at which these investigations should be repeated is not well understood, although many investigators suggest that they should be repeated annually for 3 years and then periodically thereafter.

TREATMENT

There are few prospective, well-designed trials to inform treatment of IIMs. The goals of treatment center around improving muscle strength and endurance as well as management of extramuscular features, including rashes, ILD, and dysphagia. Treatment of IIMs typically starts with corticosteroids, at doses of 1 mg/kg, and is tapered slowly once muscle enzymes have normalized. In severe disease, consideration can be given to treatment with high-dose intravenous (IV) methylprednisolone (1 g IV daily for 3 days). When patients fail to respond fully to corticosteroids, or when a steroid-sparing approach is warranted, other immunosuppressive agents often are added. Frequently, methotrexate and/or azathioprine are used in combination with corticosteroids. Methotrexate can be administered either orally or subcutaneously, at dosages of up to 25 mg per week. Methotrexate often is avoided in patients with, or at high-risk of, developing ILD, due to difficulties in discriminating methotrexate pneumonitis from myositis associated lung disease. As such, azathioprine (2–3 mg/kg per day) may be preferred in patients with ILD. As with methotrexate, evidence for its benefit in the management of myositis, is based largely on small retrospective data.[20,21] Mycophenolate mofetil, which inhibits T-cell and B-cell proliferation, increasingly is used in the management of IIMs. It typically is dosed at 2000 mg/d to 3000 mg/d, for patients with refractory IIMs and may have a use particularly in patients with myositis associated ILD.[22,23] Calcineurin inhibitors (cyclosporin and tacrolimus) also have been used successfully in refractory cases of myositis and again may be useful in the management of ILD.[24] Cyclophosphamide typically is reserved for patients with severe, refractory disease or rapidly progressive ILD. Rituximab was studied in a large, double-blind, randomized controlled trial that enrolled patients with myositis refractory to steroids and at least 1 immunosuppressive agent. Although the trial did not meet its primary outcome, 83% of patients met the definition of improvement and rituximab were shown to have a steroid-sparing effect.[25] In this trial, the presence of antibodies to Mi-2 or Jo-1 was predictive of response to treatment. Janus kinase reduces interferon signaling, which has been shown to be up-regulated in DM. Tofacitinib has been shown in case reports and small series to be beneficial in the management of refractory skin lesions of DM as well as in refractory myositis and ILD.[26–28] Other biologic agents, including tocilizumab and abatacept, have shown promise in small series and larger trials are ongoing to better define their use in management of myositis.[29,30]

Intravenous immunoglobulin (IVIG) often is used as an adjunctive therapy in the management of IIMs. The exact mechanism by which IVIG exerts an immunomodulatory effect is not well understood, although it has been used successfully in management of immune-mediated processes. Typically administered as a monthly infusion, at a dose 2 g/kg (divided over 2 consecutive days), this treatment often is used in combination with other immunosuppressive agents and/or corticosteroids. It also may be a useful agent in the management of patients with concomitant malignancy or infections. IVIG also has been shown beneficial in the management of dysphagia in myositis.[31]

Although many agents have shown promise in the management of IIMs, there are few data from randomized controlled trials to inform treatment. Revised classification criteria and well-defined outcome measures hopefully will facilitate efforts for future randomized controlled trials on the management IIMs. Currently, most patients have residual muscle weakness, reduced muscular endurance, and a reduced quality of life, despite medical treatment.

EXERCISE

Previously, exercise was not recommended in patients with active IIMs due to concerns of potentiating muscle damage. Recently, several trials have demonstrated the safety and efficacy of exercise in the management of inflammatory myopathies. Functional outcomes, including muscle strength and improvement in quality of life, have been demonstrated in well-designed trials investigating the safety and efficacy of resistance and aerobic exercise in patients with active and new-onset PM/DM, without any indicators of increased muscle inflammation.[32] A randomized controlled trial demonstrated the benefits of exercise in patients with established PM/DM, showing improvements in muscle performance, maximum oxygen consumption (Vo_{2max}), and disease activity after a 12-week supervised endurance exercise program.[33] Furthermore, immunohistochemical analysis of muscle biopsies taken before and after an endurance training program demonstrated downregulation of genes related to inflammation, fibrosis, endoplasmic reticulum stress, and up-regulation of genes related involved in muscle growth and changes in mRNA and proteins associated with capillary growth.[34] In patients with IBM, a 12-week program of resistance training demonstrated lesser declines in muscle function relative to those in the control group.[35] Exercise is proved as an important component of the management of patients with IIMs and may help with improvement or preservation of muscle strength and improvements in endurance and quality of life. Contrary to previous dogma, exercise has been shown to be safe in all types and stages of IIMs.

Prognosis/Outcomes

Although the outcomes of patients with IIMs have improved with corticosteroid and immunosuppressive therapies, it remains a disorder characterized by significantly increased mortality and morbidity. Patients with IIMs reported poorer health as measured by the 36-item short form health survey (SF-36), compared with the general population.[36] Patients with IIMs have a 3-fold increase risk of death relative to the general population.[37] The main causes of death are malignancies and infection.[38] Factors associated with a worse prognosis include cancer-associated myositis, DM, ILD, overlap myositis, and elevated acute phase reactants at presentation. Five-year survival rates in a US cohort were 90% in IIM patients without ILD and 81% with ILD, although geographic variation in mortality exists.[39]

SUMMARY

IIMs are autoimmune disorders that can affect all ages and are characterized by a spectrum of clinical manifestations, the most common of which is skeletal muscle weakness. Several MSAs have been identified and may help to inform treatment and direct the evaluation for extramuscular features. As a multisystemic disorder, a thoughtful approach taking into consideration clinical, serologic, and histologic data is required to develop a patient-specific management strategy. Treatment remains suboptimal in many cases and, owing to the rarity of these disorders, is based primarily on small series because there a few randomized controlled trials to inform management of IIMs.

REFERENCES

1. Svensson J, Arkema EV, Lundberg IE, et al. Incidence and prevalence of idiopathic inflammatory myopathies in Sweden: a nationwide population-based study. Rheumatology (Oxford) 2017;56(5):802–10.
2. Fiorentino D, Chung L, Zwerner J, et al. The mucocutaneous and systemic phenotype of dermatomyositis patients with antibodies to MDA5 (CADM-140): a retrospective study. J Am Acad Dermatol 2011;65(1):25–34.
3. Nakashima R, Imura Y, Kobayashi S, et al. The RIG-I-like receptor IFIH1/MDA5 is a dermatomyositis-specific autoantigen identified by the anti-CADM-140 antibody. Rheumatology (Oxford) 2010;49(3):433–40.
4. Sato S, Hoshino K, Satoh T, et al. RNA helicase encoded by melanoma differentiation-associated gene 5 is a major autoantigen in patients with clinically amyopathic dermatomyositis: Association with rapidly progressive interstitial lung disease. Arthritis Rheum 2009;60(7):2193–200.
5. Mendez EP, Lipton R, Ramsey-Goldman R, et al. US incidence of juvenile dermatomyositis, 1995-1998: results from the National Institute of Arthritis and Musculoskeletal and Skin Diseases Registry. Arthritis Rheum 2003;49(3):300–5.
6. Betteridge Z, McHugh N. Myositis-specific autoantibodies: an important tool to support diagnosis of myositis. J Intern Med 2016;280(1):8–23.
7. Cox FM, Titulaer MJ, Sont JK, et al. A 12-year follow-up in sporadic inclusion body myositis: an end stage with major disabilities. Brain 2011;134(Pt 11): 3167–75.
8. Day J, Patel S, Limaye V. The role of magnetic resonance imaging techniques in evaluation and management of the idiopathic inflammatory myopathies. Semin Arthritis Rheum 2017;46(5):642–9.
9. Chahin N, Engel AG. Correlation of muscle biopsy, clinical course, and outcome in PM and sporadic IBM. Neurology 2008;70(6):418–24.
10. Koenig M, Fritzler MJ, Targoff IN, et al. Heterogeneity of autoantibodies in 100 patients with autoimmune myositis: insights into clinical features and outcomes. Arthritis Res Ther 2007;9(4):R78.
11. Lega JC, Fabien N, Reynaud Q, et al. The clinical phenotype associated with myositis-specific and associated autoantibodies: a meta-analysis revisiting the so-called antisynthetase syndrome. Autoimmun Rev 2014;13(9):883–91.
12. Aggarwal R, Cassidy E, Fertig N, et al. Patients with non-Jo-1 anti-tRNA-synthetase autoantibodies have worse survival than Jo-1 positive patients. Ann Rheum Dis 2014;73(1):227–32.
13. Fiorentino DF, Chung LS, Christopher-Stine L, et al. Most patients with cancer-associated dermatomyositis have antibodies to nuclear matrix protein NXP-2 or transcription intermediary factor 1gamma. Arthritis Rheum 2013;65(11):2954–62.
14. Tiniakou E, Mammen AL. Idiopathic inflammatory myopathies and malignancy: a comprehensive review. Clin Rev Allergy Immunol 2017;52(1):20–33.
15. Allenbach Y, Drouot L, Rigolet A, et al. Anti-HMGCR autoantibodies in European patients with autoimmune necrotizing myopathies: inconstant exposure to statin. Medicine (Baltimore) 2014;93(3):150–7.
16. Larman HB, Salajegheh M, Nazareno R, et al. Cytosolic 5'-nucleotidase 1A autoimmunity in sporadic inclusion body myositis. Ann Neurol 2013;73(3):408–18.

17. Pluk H, van Hoeve BJ, van Dooren SH, et al. Autoantibodies to cytosolic 5'-nucleotidase 1A in inclusion body myositis. Ann Neurol 2013;73(3):397–407.
18. Andras C, Ponyi A, Constantin T, et al. Dermatomyositis and polymyositis associated with malignancy: a 21-year retrospective study. J Rheumatol 2008;35(3):438–44.
19. Hill CL, Zhang Y, Sigurgeirsson B, et al. Frequency of specific cancer types in dermatomyositis and polymyositis: a population-based study. Lancet 2001;357(9250):96–100.
20. Joffe MM, Love LA, Leff RL, et al. Drug therapy of the idiopathic inflammatory myopathies: predictors of response to prednisone, azathioprine, and methotrexate and a comparison of their efficacy. Am J Med 1993;94(4):379–87.
21. Bunch TW. Prednisone and azathioprine for polymyositis: long-term followup. Arthritis Rheum 1981;24(1):45–8.
22. Huapaya JA, Silhan L, Pinal-Fernandez I, et al. Long-term treatment with azathioprine and mycophenolate mofetil for myositis-related interstitial lung disease. Chest 2019;156(5):896–906.
23. Pisoni CN, Cuadrado MJ, Khamashta MA, et al. Mycophenolate mofetil treatment in resistant myositis. Rheumatology (Oxford) 2007;46(3):516–8.
24. Oddis CV, Sciurba FC, Elmagd KA, et al. Tacrolimus in refractory polymyositis with interstitial lung disease. Lancet 1999;353(9166):1762–3.
25. Oddis CV, Reed AM, Aggarwal R, et al. Rituximab in the treatment of refractory adult and juvenile dermatomyositis and adult polymyositis: a randomized, placebo-phase trial. Arthritis Rheum 2013;65(2):314–24.
26. Paik JJ, Christopher-Stine L. A case of refractory dermatomyositis responsive to tofacitinib. Semin Arthritis Rheum 2017;46(4):e19.
27. Moghadam-Kia S, Charlton D, Aggarwal R, et al. Management of refractory cutaneous dermatomyositis: potential role of Janus kinase inhibition with tofacitinib. Rheumatology (Oxford) 2019;58(6):1011–5.
28. Kurasawa K, Arai S, Namiki Y, et al. Tofacitinib for refractory interstitial lung diseases in anti-melanoma differentiation-associated 5 gene antibody-positive dermatomyositis. Rheumatology (Oxford) 2018;57(12):2114–9.
29. Narazaki M, Hagihara K, Shima Y, et al. Therapeutic effect of tocilizumab on two patients with polymyositis. Rheumatology (Oxford) 2011;50(7):1344–6.
30. Musuruana JL, Cavallasca JA. Abatacept for treatment of refractory polymyositis. Joint Bone Spine 2011;78(4):431–2.
31. Marie I, Menard JF, Hatron PY, et al. Intravenous immunoglobulins for steroid-refractory esophageal involvement related to polymyositis and dermatomyositis: a series of 73 patients. Arthritis Care Res (Hoboken) 2010;62(12):1748–55.
32. Alexanderson H. Exercise in Myositis. Curr Treatm Opt Rheumatol 2018;4(4):289–98.
33. Alemo Munters L, Dastmalchi M, Andgren V, et al. Improvement in health and possible reduction in disease activity using endurance exercise in patients with established polymyositis and dermatomyositis: a multicenter randomized controlled trial with a 1-year open extension followup. Arthritis Care Res (Hoboken) 2013;65(12):1959–68.
34. Munters LA, Loell I, Ossipova E, et al. Endurance exercise improves molecular pathways of aerobic metabolism in patients with myositis. Arthritis Rheumatol 2016;68(7):1738–50.
35. Jorgensen AN, Aagaard P, Frandsen U, et al. Blood-flow restricted resistance training in patients with sporadic inclusion body myositis: a randomized controlled trial. Scand J Rheumatol 2018;47(5):400–9.

36. Sultan SM, Ioannou Y, Moss K, et al. Outcome in patients with idiopathic inflammatory myositis: morbidity and mortality. Rheumatology (Oxford) 2002; 41(1):22–6.
37. Dobloug GC, Svensson J, Lundberg IE, et al. Mortality in idiopathic inflammatory myopathy: results from a Swedish nationwide population-based cohort study. Ann Rheum Dis 2018;77(1):40–7.
38. Nuno-Nuno L, Joven BE, Carreira PE, et al. Mortality and prognostic factors in idiopathic inflammatory myositis: a retrospective analysis of a large multicenter cohort of Spain. Rheumatol Int 2017;37(11):1853–61.
39. Johnson C, Pinal-Fernandez I, Parikh R, et al. Assessment of mortality in autoimmune myositis with and without associated interstitial lung disease. Lung 2016; 194(5):733–7.

Osteoporosis Diagnosis and Management

Richard Pope, MPAS, PA-C, DFAAPA, CPAAPA[a,b,c,d,]*, Joan Doback, MHP, PA-C[b,e,f]

KEYWORDS

- Osteoporosis • Osteopenia • Low bone density • Bone Mineral Density (BMD)
- Fragility fracture • DXA • FRAX • Male osteoporosis

KEY POINTS

- Postmenopausal osteoporosis is a growing public health problem and is a common condition associated with fractures that occur after minimal or, in some cases, no trauma.
- It is important to recognize this condition because it can be diagnosed and prevented before fractures occur.
- Osteoporosis is a chronic disease that affects all ethnicity groups and is more common in women than in men, is under-recognized and undertreated, and requires management throughout life.
- There are several validated tools that assist in fracture risk assessment.
- There are many universal recommendations for healthy bones and medications approved by the US Food and Drug Administration that use different mechanisms for prevention and treatment.

INTRODUCTION

Osteoporosis (OP) is the most common bone disease in humans and has become a major public health problem. It is characterized by low bone mass, deterioration of bone tissue and disruption of bone architecture, compromised bone strength, and an increase in the risk of fracture. It is a silent disease until it leads to fracture. OP exacts both an enormous financial and human toll. It is estimated that 10.2 million people in the United States have OP, and another 43 million have osteopenia or low bone mass. The cost of treating osteoporotic fractures in the United States is estimated to increase to $25.3 billion by 2025[1] **(Fig. 1).**

[a] Department of Rheumatology, Nuvance Health, Danbury, CT, USA; [b] Department of Physician Assistant Studies, Quinnipiac University, North Haven, CT, USA; [c] University of Bridgeport, Bridgeport, CT, USA; [d] Yale University School of Medicine, New Haven, CT, USA; [e] Department of Orthopedics, Waterbury Health, Waterbury, CT, USA; [f] Department of Public Health and Community Medicine, Tufts University, Boston, MA, USA
* Corresponding author.
E-mail address: Pop5rjhjc@aol.com

Physician Assist Clin 6 (2021) 111–133
https://doi.org/10.1016/j.cpha.2020.09.009

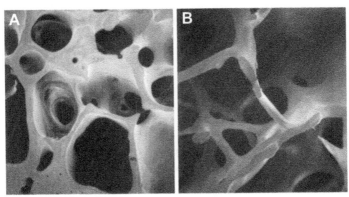

Fig. 1. (*A*) Normal versus (*B*) OP. (*From* Chabner, DE. Musculoskeletal System. The Language of Medicine, Twelfth Edition. Philadelphia: Elsevier, 2021; with permission.)

There are many common medical conditions that are encountered in primary care that are associated with or contribute to OP. A partial list is in **Box 1**.

HISTORY
Medical History

A thorough medical history and review of systems obtained by having a thoughtful detailed discussion with the patient, and often using a simple intake questionnaire,

---

Box 1
Common medical conditions associated with OP

- Endocrine disorders
  - Diabetes type 1 and type 2
  - Hyperthyroidism, including long-standing overtreatment for thyroid replacement
  - Hyperparathyroidism
  - Hypogonadism

- Nutritional and gastrointestinal conditions
  - Crohn's disease
  - Malabsorption syndromes (celiac disease, gastrointestinal surgery including resection/bypass)
  - Anorexia nervosa
  - Calcium deficiency
  - Vitamin D deficiency

- Other
  - Chronic obstructive pulmonary disease
  - AIDS/human immunodeficiency virus infection
  - Ankylosing spondylitis
  - Rheumatoid arthritis
  - Hypercalciuria
  - Major depression
  - Renal insufficiency or failure
  - Thalassemia
  - Systemic mastocytosis
  - Myeloma and some cancers
  - Immobilization

can guide further workup. Specific risk factors that may identify contributing causes of OP and that will be essential in the assessment of fracture risk are found in **Box 2**. The history should include both the past medical history and a personal OP history. Personal OP history elements are found in **Box 3**.

Surgical History

The past surgical history should pay close attention to hysterectomy, oophorectomy, bariatric surgery, and thyroid or parathyroid surgery.

Family History

A parental history of fracture has been associated with a modest but significantly increased risk of any fracture, osteoporotic fracture, and hip fracture.[2,3]

Social History

A social history should question a patient's living situation, including independence or need for assistance, use of assistive devices when ambulating, and any falls that have occurred in the past year. A provider should also inquire about a patient's diet, including protein intake, calcium and vitamin D intake, and history of eating disorders. Exercise routine, and a history of cigarette smoking and alcohol use are important. Obtaining a list of current medications from the patient is important and can uncover medications that contribute to declining bone health (**Box 4**).

PHYSICAL EXAMINATION AND WORKUP

Measurement of weight and height are imperative in the assessment of bone health. Compared with women who weighed more than 73.3 kg (161 pounds), women who weighed less than 57.8 kg (127 pounds) were about 2 times more likely to have fractures of the hip, pelvis, and ribs.[4] The accuracy of the height measurement is critical and should be performed preferably on a wall-mounted stadiometer and compared with previous height and height at age 20. Loss of more than 1.5 inches (3.8 cm) signals the possibility of vertebral compression fractures (VCF).[5] In this case, consideration should be given to a vertebral fracture assessment (VFA) or to a lateral thoracolumbar radiograph to assess for compression fractures. The evaluation of posture and the finding of thoracic kyphosis will further the suspicion of VCF. Eliciting tenderness of the spine on percussion or palpation may also indicate VCF.

Box 2 **Risk factors for OP**
Age
Sex
History of previous fractures
History of parental hip fracture
Cigarette smoking
Alcohol consumption of 3 or more units daily
Use of glucocorticoid medication
History of rheumatoid arthritis or other secondary cause of OP

Box 3
Elements of personal OP history

Age

Height

Weight

A gynecologic history of early onset of menopause and the use of hormone replacement therapy after menopause

A specific history of fragility fracture in adulthood as defined by a fracture of any bone except finger, toes, and skull that was sustained from a fall from standing height

Past treatment of OP detailed along with the duration and side effects of medications

A history of more than 2 falls in the past year

An assessment of fall risk is essential because most fragility fractures are due to falls. A comprehensive screening and assessment of the patient's fall risk can be located through the US Centers for Disease Control and Prevention, where they have developed an algorithm that details each step of physical evaluation for falls and guides interventions based on level of risk. The Stopping Elderly Accidents, Deaths, and Injuries (STEADI) algorithm can be found at https://www.cdc.gov/steadi/.

Laboratory Evaluation

A cost-effective basic laboratory panel that would eliminate the most common causes of secondary OP should include a complete blood count, serum parathyroid hormone (PTH), 24-hour urine collection for calcium and creatinine levels, comprehensive metabolic panel, thyroid-stimulating hormone, and a serum 25 hydroxyvitamin D level.[6]

Bone Mineral Density

The gold standard for evaluating bone mineral density (BMD) is the dual energy x-ray absorptiometry (DXA) scan. The BMD of an area is expressed in terms of grams of mineral per square centimeter scanned (g/cm^2) and as a relationship to either of 2 reference populations. When compared with the BMD of an age-, sex-, and ethnicity-matched reference population, a Z-score is reported. When compared

---

Box 4
Medications that contribute to declining bone health

Antiepileptics

Aromatase inhibitors

Chemotherapy and immunosuppressants

DepoProvera

Glucocorticoids

Gonadotropin-releasing hormone agonists

Data from Watts NB, Bilezikian JP, Camacho PM, et al. American Association of Clinical Endocrinologists Medical Guidelines for Clinical Practice for the diagnosis and treatment of postmenopausal osteoporosis. Endocr Pract. 2010;16 Suppl 3(Suppl 3):1-37. https://doi.org/10.4158/ep.16.s3.1.

---

with a young adult reference population of the same sex, a T-score is reported. T-scores are used in the evaluation of postmenopausal women, and Z-scores are only used and recommended for premenopausal women. Z-scores of –2 or more standard deviations below the mean are considered "below the expected range for age"[7] (**Table 1**).

FRAX Calculator

FRAX is a validated tool used to calculate the 10-year probability of a hip fracture and the 10-year probability of a major osteoporotic fracture (defined as clinical vertebral, hip, forearm, or proximal humerus fracture), taking into account certain clinical risk factors and femoral neck BMD when available. FRAX is best applied to those with T-scores between –1.0 standard deviations and –2.5 standard deviations and helps clinicians to identify individuals who would benefit from treatment. The FRAX calculator recommends postmenopausal women or men over the age of 50 with a 10-year probability of a hip fracture of 3% or higher or a 10-year probability of a major OP-related fracture of 20% or higher based on the US-adapted World Health Organization (WHO) algorithm be considered for treatment with medications approved by the US Food and Drug Administration (FDA).[8] The FRAX calculator can be found at: https://www.sheffield.ac.uk/FRAX.

Additional Tools for Evaluation

VFA, trabecular bone score (TBS), and bone turnover markers are all helpful in further evaluating for risk of fracture. Some DXA machines have add on software for VFA and TBS. If VFA is not available in your area and if there has been height loss of 1.5 inches in a postmenopausal female or 2.5 inches in a male, then a simple spinal radiograph can be ordered with attention to T5 through L4 while alerting the radiologist to look for compression fractures. TBS performs texture measurements of lumbar vertebra related to trabecular microarchitecture. TBS is an independent risk for fracture that is particularly sensitive in assessing patients with diabetes and patients with glucocorticoid-induced OP. Only recently developed, its use is limited owing to a

Table 1
WHO definitions of OP based on BMD

Classification	BMD	T Score
Normal	Within 1 SD of the mean level for a young adult reference population	T score at –1.0 and above
Low bone mass (osteopenia)	Between 1 and 2.5 SD below that of the mean level for a young adult reference population	T score between –1.0 and –2.5
OP	2.5 or more below that of the mean level for a young adult reference population	T score at or below –2.5
Severe or established OP	2.5 or more below that of the mean level for a young adult reference population with fractures	T score at or below –2.5 with one or more fractures

Abbreviation: SD, standard deviation.
From Kanis JA on behalf of the World Health Organization Scientific Group. Technical Report. World Health Organization Collaborating Centre for Metabolic Bone Diseases, University of Sheffield; UK: 2007. 2007. Assessment of osteoporosis at the primary health-care level; with permission.

lack of equipped DXA machines. Bone turnover markers continue to be an emerging tool in the assessment and management of bone health. Becoming more widely used, there is a recognized wide variation in their results and continue to be used more in research than clinical practice. Serum carboxy-terminal collagen crosslinks for antiresorptive medication compliance and *N*-terminal propeptide of type 1 collagen for PTH analogs are now recommended as the go-to markers by the International Osteoporosis Foundation (**Fig. 2**).

INDICATIONS FOR TREATMENT

Expanded criteria recommend that postmenopausal women and men age 50 and older presenting with the following should be considered for treatment:

- T-score of −2.5 or less at the femoral neck, total hip, or lumbar spine.
- A low trauma hip fracture (regardless of bone density)
- Fracture of vertebrae, proximal humerus, pelvis, or wrist in a setting of osteopenia (T-score between −1.0 and −2.5)
- Low bone mass (T-score between −1.0 and −2.5 at the femoral neck or lumbar spine) and a 10-year probability of a hip fracture of 3% or higher or a 10-year probability of a major OP-related fracture of 20% or higher based on the US-adapted WHO algorithm[9]

Universal Recommendations

Nutrition
A balanced diet rich in low-fat dairy products, fruits, vegetables, and protein is of lifetime importance for bone health. Of the more specific considerations of nutrition for bone health, calcium and vitamin D are most important.

Calcium
The National Osteoporosis Foundation recommends that postmenopausal women consume 1200 mg/d of calcium.[10] It has not been proven that intake of higher than

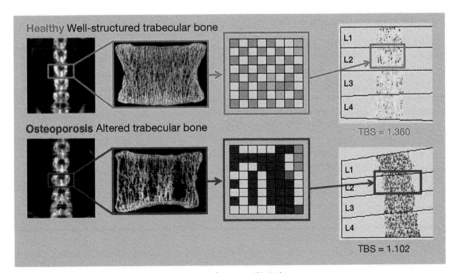

Fig. 2. Trabecular bone score. (*Courtesy of* Mayo Clinic.)

1200 mg/d confers benefit; in fact, some literature points to intake of more than 1500 mg/d may increase the risk of developing cardiovascular disease, stroke, and kidney stones.[11,12] Consensus of bone health experts concluded that the current evidence suggests that dietary calcium may be preferred over supplemental calcium and that a daily total calcium should not exceed 1500 mg/d.[13] For those patients who are unable to increase their calcium intake in their diets, calcium supplementation should be recommended to reach goal intake. Patients with a history of hypercalcemia would not want to use supplemental calcium. In addition, in patients with a history of proven calcium oxalate kidney stones, maximizing dietary calcium is preferred (**Box 5**).

Vitamin D

Vitamin D, although commonly referred to as a "vitamin," is a prohormone that is produced in the epidermis of the skin during interaction with UVB rays of sunlight. Dietary sources of vitamin D are limited to few food sources such as fatty fish and foods fortified with vitamin D, including dairy products, orange juice, soy milk, and cereals. Therefore, for most people, taking a vitamin D_2 (ergocalciferol) or vitamin D_3 (cholecalciferol) supplement is the most reliable means of ensuring adequate intake. **Box 6** provides a list of risks for vitamin D deficiency or insufficiency.

Based on evidence that secondary hyperparathyroidism is increasingly common at 25(OH)D levels of less than 30 ng/mL[14] and that calcium absorption efficiency plateaus at vitamin D at approximately 32 ng/mL, consensus bone health expert opinion holds that sufficiency be defined as 20 ng/mL, with the majority favoring 29 to 32 ng/mL.[15,16] The National Osteoporosis Foundation recommends a daily intake of 800 to 1000 international units of vitamin D for adults age 50 years and older. Serum 25(OH)D levels should be measured in patients who are at risk of deficiency. Supplementation should be recommended in amounts sufficient to bring the serum vitamin D level to about 30 ng/mL.

A meta-analysis (DiPART) of 12 randomized clinical trials found that a significant fracture reduction was achieved with higher vitamin D doses of 700 to 800 IU daily coupled with 1000 mg of elemental calcium for nonvertebral, vertebral, and hip fractures.[17]

Exercise

A regular routine of weight-bearing exercise, muscle-strengthening exercises, and balance training should be recommended to patients of all ages. Continued habits of exercise have been shown to improve strength, agility, posture, and balance. It is necessary to strengthen the extensor muscles of the back, hip flexors and extensors, thigh, upper arm, and forearm to avoid the typical osteoporotic fractures. Among women age 75 or older, muscle-strengthening and balance exercises are shown to decrease the risk of falls and subsequent injury by 75%.[18] Exercise induced

Box 5
Estimating daily dietary sources of calcium
Milk 300 mg/glass
Almond or soy milk 450 mg/glass
Cheese 200 mg/1 0unce
Yogurt 300 mg/cup
Broccoli 172 mg/cup

Box 6
Risk for vitamin D deficiency and insufficiency

Patients who use sunblock with an SPF of 8 or greater will block 97.5% of the UVB rays

Older patients because of renal insufficiency, their reduced mobility and consequent decreased exposure to sunshine and the decreasing capacity of the skin to synthesize vitamin D with age

People with darker skin pigmentation

People who spend little time outdoors owing to variability in skin activation and synthesis of vitamin D

People who live in the northern latitudes with weak UV light, especially in the fall and winter

---

improvements in lumbar spine and femoral neck BMD could reduce fracture risk by approximately 10%.[19]

Smoking cessation

It is well-documented that cigarette smoking is deleterious to overall health and more specifically to skeletal health. Smokers tend to lose bone more rapidly, have a lower bone mass, and undergo menopause 2 years earlier than nonsmokers.[20] A meta-analysis suggested that the risk of hip fracture is also increased in smokers.[21]

Alcohol consumption

Women who drink alcohol should be advised to drink moderately and should be educated as to alcohol intake quantity. One unit of alcohol is 12 oz of beer, 4 oz of wine, or 1 oz of liquor. Three cohorts totaling more than 11,000 women showed that more than 2 alcohol units a day is associated with an increased risk of osteoporotic fracture.[22]

Fall prevention

Falls are the leading cause of injury and injury-related deaths among adults aged 65 and older. Falls are also the precipitating event in almost 90% of all appendicular fractures, including hip fractures.[23] Beyond the physical injuries associated with falling, there are often serious psychological consequences associated with falling with a cascade from fear of subsequent falls leading to becoming less active, which further leads to physical decline, social isolation, and feelings of helplessness.[24] A multifaceted approach to fall prevention has shown to be valuable. Fall prevention steps are listed in **Box 7**.

Box 7
Fall prevention steps

Muscle-strengthening exercise and balance training with physical therapy.

Home safety evaluation to reduce fall hazards inside and outside the home.

Limiting or eliminating benzodiazepines, antidepressants, and neuroleptic drugs.

Annual ophthalmologic and hearing evaluations.

PHARMACOLOGIC MANAGEMENT

As more FDA-approved medications with different mechanisms of action come on the market, it becomes important to know each category of medication, its benefits, and its side effect profile. Patients often can come with preconceived fears of side effects and it is important for practitioners to possess accurate information to dispel these.

Estrogen or Hormone Therapies

Treatment with either estrogen or hormone therapy should be reserved for those with vasomotor symptoms and vulvovaginal atrophy associated with menopause and who are less than 60 years of age. Both estrogen and hormone therapy (hormone therapy for those who have not had a hysterectomy) can prevent bone density loss and prevent fracture.[25]

The Endocrine Society suggests estrogen or hormone therapy under certain conditions.[25]

- Patients who cannot take bisphosphonates or denosumab
- Patients under the age of 60 or 10 years past menopause
- Patients with vasomotor or climacteric symptoms

Selective Estrogen Modulators

Raloxifene, a selective modulator of estrogen, is FDA approved for the prevention and treatment of OP in postmenopausal women and has a second indication for risk reduction of invasive breast cancer in postmenopausal women with a risk of breast cancer owing to family history.[26–29] Raloxifene does not decrease the risk of coronary heart disease.[30] It does decrease the risk of incident vertebral fractures by about 30% to 40% in patients with a prior vertebral fracture and approximately 55% in patients without a prior vertebral fracture. There is a lack of evidence to support reduction in hip and nonvertebral fracture.

Bisphosphonates

Bisphosphonates are often given as first-line agents to decrease bone breakdown. Mechanistically, they adhere to bone, interfering with osteoclastic function and thereby reduce bone turnover, which leads to increased mineralization over time. Bisphosphonates can be given both orally (alendronate, risedronate, and ibandronate) and intravenously (IV) (ibandronate and zoledronic acid). Three of the 4 (alendronate, risedronate, and zoledronic acid) commonly used bisphosphonates have evidence for broad-spectrum antifracture efficacy.[31–34] Ibandronate did not show fracture protection for hip and nonvertebral fractures in phase III trials.

Bisphosphonates improve BMD in the first 3 to 5 years after initiation; however, the duration of treatment with these agents ranges from 3 to 10 years, depending on the severity of the disease, patient risk profile, and expert opinion.[35] Contraindications to oral bisphosphonates include the ability to comply with dosing instructions, which requires taking the medication after a prolonged fast and 30 minutes before other medications, food, or beverages other than water.[36,37] Patients with active esophageal and gastrointestinal diseases such as achalasia, stricture, esophageal dysmotility, Barrett's esophagus, severe gastroesophageal reflux disease, gastric bypass, Crohn's disease, or ulcerative colitis should not receive oral bisphosphonates. Other side effects include postdosing myalgias, arthralgias, and, less commonly, fever and hypocalcemia. Oral and IV bisphosphonates are contraindicated in patients with decreased renal function, specifically, those with a glomerular filtration rate of less than 30 mL/min for risedronate and ibandronate or less than 35 mL/min for alendronate and zoledronic acid.[38] Rare occurrences of osteonecrosis of the jaw (ONJ) and atypical femoral fracture have occurred.

Side effects of IV zoledronic acid include an acute phase reaction of postinfusion myalgias, arthralgias, headache, and fever. They are usually mild and transient over 1 to 3 days, but can be seen up to 14 days later. These side effects occurred in phase III studies in approximately 15% of patients.[39,40] Subsequent annual dosing showed an approximate 50% decrease in these acute phase reactions. All patients should be encouraged to be well hydrated before the infusion and throughout the day of the infusion. Acetaminophen is recommended to treat postinfusion reactions and can be given ahead of the infusion prophylactically. Acute renal failure has been seen with IV zoledronic acid.[41]

Rank Ligand Inhibitor

There is presently one rank ligand (RANKL) inhibitor, denosumab, approved by the FDA for prevention and treatment of OP. Denosumab is a fully humanized monoclonal antibody and is given as a 60-mg subcutaneous injection every 6 months. In pivotal trials including 7808 women over 3 years, denosumab showed a broad protection from fractures in the spine, hip, and nonvertebral sites. The indications for denosumab include:

- Treatment of postmenopausal women at high risk for fracture.
- To increase bone mass in men with OP who are at high risk for fracture.
- To treat glucocorticoid induced OP in both men and women at high risk for fracture.
- To increase bone mass in men at high risk for fracture receiving androgen deprivation therapy for nonmetastatic prostate cancer.
- To increase bone mass in women who are at high risk for fracture receiving adjuvant aromatase inhibitor therapy for breast cancer.

Denosumab is a potent antiresorptive agent and decreases vertebral fractures by 68%, hip fractures by 40%, and nonvertebral fractures by 20% at 3 years.[42,43] Denosumab may cause or exacerbate hypocalcemia, and therefore hypocalcemia must be corrected before treatment. Safety profiles are like those of bisphosphonates and placebo. Long-term extension trials have shown no new safety concerns, although a theoretic infection risk exists with RANKL inhibition.

Discontinuation of denosumab treatment is associated with rapid bone loss that may result in multiple vertebral fractures, especially in patients with a prior vertebral fracture.[44] It has been shown that denosumab followed by a bisphosphonate preserves bone mass.[45]

Two rare side effects can occur with the long-term use of bisphosphonates, RANKL inhibitors, and sclerostin inhibitors but are not seen with PTH analogs. The first is osteonecrosis of the jaw (ONJ), also known as medication-related ONJ in the dental literature. Statistically reviewed, medication-related ONJ has a risk of between 1 in 10,000 and 1 in 100,000 patient-years in the OP population.[46] In a patient treated for OP, the most likely scenario for ONJ occurs after dental extraction. There is a higher incidence of ONJ in the cancer population owing to more frequent and higher dosing of bisphosphonates for cancer-related effects. In 2011, the American Dental Association published a statement agreeing that the benefits of OP therapy outweighed the risks of ONJ[47] (**Fig. 3**).

The second rare side effect associated with long term treatment with antiresorptive medications is atypical femoral fracture. This is a transverse fracture starting from the lateral cortex below the lesser trochanter in the subtrochanteric region or

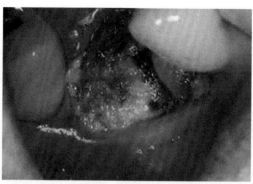

Fig. 3. Osteonecrosis of the Jaw. (*From* Wikimedia Images. Coronation Dental Specialty Group Available at: https://en.wikipedia.org/wiki/Medication-related_osteonecrosis_of_the_jaw#/media/File:Stage_2_MRONJ.jpg.)

diaphysis. The fracture has a general transverse orientation, a lack of comminution, localized cortical thickening, and may have a medial spike. The mechanism is not clear, but may be due to oversuppression of bone that can occur with the long-term use of nitrogen-containing bisphosphonates (alendronate, risedronate, zole-dronic acid, ibandronate, and pamidronate) and has been seen with the use of denosumab.

In about 70% to 75% of patients, there is a prodromal thigh pain that occurs weeks to months before the fracture.[48] Evaluation of a patient with anterior thigh or hip pain who is on bisphosphonates should include a full-length femoral radiograph looking for atypical femoral fracture and in some instances an MRI may be needed to identify the fracture (**Fig. 4**).

Parathyroid Analogs

Teriparatide is an FDA approved treatment for those at high risk of fracture:

- Postmenopausal women and men at high risk for fracture.
- Risk associated with sustained systemic glucocorticoid therapy.
- For patients who have failed or are intolerant to other available OP therapy.
- For men with hypogonadism.

The dose is 20 μg/d subcutaneous designed as a self-injection for 18 to 24 months. Teriparatide decreases risk of vertebral fractures by 65% to 73%, hip fractures by 56%, and nonvertebral fragility fractures by 38% to 53% in patients with OP, after an average of 18 months of therapy.[49]

Abaloparatide is a synthetic analog of PTH-related peptide, and is FDA approved for postmenopausal women at high risk of fracture, defined as multiple risk factors for fracture, or who have failed or are intolerant to other available OP therapies. It is not yet approved for men. The dose is 80 μg self-subcutaneous injection monthly for 18 to 24 months.

Abaloparatide decreases the risk of new vertebral fractures by about 86% and non-vertebral fractures by about 43% in postmenopausal women with OP, after an average of 18 months of therapy.[50] In an extension study after 18 months, the addition of 6 months of oral alendronate for a total of up to 24 months of treatment resulted in a relative risk reduction of radiographic spine fractures by 87%, nonvertebral fractures by 52%, and major osteoporotic fractures by 58%.[51]

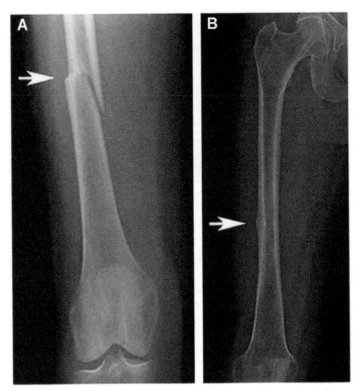

Fig. 4. Radiographic views of (*A*) an atypical femoral fracture that occurred spontaneously in a woman after 6 years of treatment with a bisphosphonate and (*B*) an incomplete atypical femoral fracture with cortical thickening that presented as thigh pain. (*From* Khan AA, Kaiser S. Atypical femoral fracture. CMAJ. 2017;189(14):E542. https://doi.org/10.1503/cmaj. 160450; with permission.)

Teriparatide and abaloparatide are both contraindicated in patients with increased risk of osteosarcoma (eg, Paget's disease of bone, bone metastases, prior skeletal radiation). Since the release of teriparatide in 2002, there have been 3 reported cases of osteosarcoma worldwide, which does not exceed the incidence in the general population.[52] Additionally, patients with hypercalcemia or a history of an unexplained elevated alkaline phosphatase or skeletal malignancy should not receive either agent. Both medications may increase urinary calcium and therefore should be used with caution in patients with active or recent kidney stones because of the potential to exacerbate this condition.[53] It is common practice to use follow-on therapy after either agent using an antiresorptive such as a bisphosphonate or denosumab to maintain and further improve BMD and prevent bone loss that occurs after discontinuing.

Sclerostin Inhibitor

Romosozumab is a monoclonal antibody to sclerostin approved by the FDA for women who are at high risk for fracture. Its mechanism of action has a dual effect on bone, both increasing bone formation and decreasing breakdown. Romosozumab decreases fracture and increases BMD at the lumbar spine and total hip more than placebo, alendronate, and teriparatide in postmenopausal women with low bone mass.[54,55] In the pivotal FRAME trial, romosozumab, when compared with placebo, decreased the risk of new vertebral fractures by 73%, clinical fractures by 36%, and hip fracture by 38%.[56]

Extension studies have shown trends of BMD reversing to baseline suggesting that follow-on therapy with an antiresorptive agent such as a bisphosphonate or denosumab would maintain and continue to accrue BMD benefits.[57] FDA approval included a black box warning that it may increase risks for myocardial infarction, stroke, and cardiovascular death. It should not be taken by patients who experienced a cardiovascular or stroke event in the previous year. It may also cause hypocalcemia and has been associated with hypersensitivity reactions such as angioedema, erythema multiforme, rash, and urticaria. In the same vein as bisphosphonates and RANKL inhibitors, patients using romosozumab are at low but increased risk of ONJ and atypical femoral fractures.[58]

Fracture Liaison Service

A fracture liaison service is an established and proven method to achieve recommended standards of care for fragility fractures, including intervention for OP, secondary fracture prevention, and bone health evaluation. Fracture liaison services focus on secondary fracture prevention by identifying patients at risk for future fracture and initiating appropriate evaluation, risk assessment, education, and therapeutic interventions. The fracture liaison service is usually composed of 3 team members: the Bone Health Champion, who usually is a physician with special interest or training in OP; the Bone Health Coordinator, who is usually a physician assistant or nurse practitioner; and the Nurse Navigator.[59] The fracture liaison service aims to seamlessly transition fragility fracture patients from surgical or nonoperative orthopedic care of the fracture to long-term management of OP to treat the disease process and prevent secondary fractures. It has been proven to improve diagnosis, improve long-term treatment and to decrease morbidity in these patients.

Special Considerations: Glucocorticoid-Induced Osteoporosis

Glucocorticoids play an important role in treating many inflammatory conditions. Approximately 1% of the US population is treated with long-term glucocorticoids. Both oral and parenteral glucocorticoids have significant negative effects, including fracture and bone loss. More than 1 of 10 patients who receive long-term treatment are diagnosed with a fracture and 30% to 40% have radiographic evidence of a VCF. For patients who are on glucocorticoids, fracture incidence increases with longer term use (over 5 years), higher doses (>7.5 mg/d), older age (>55 years), female sex, and Caucasian race. The highest rate of bone loss occurs in the first 3 to 6 months; however, the decline continues more slowly with prolonged use. Glucocorticoid effects on bone are reversible when the medication is discontinued, because the BMD improves and the fracture risk declines.[60] In addition, the use of OP medications in glucocorticoid-treated patients has been shown to reduce new vertebral fractures by 43% in a Cochrane analysis of randomized controlled trials, similar to effects seen in postmenopausal OP.[61]

For the purposes of this review, glucocorticoid-induced OP will be addressed in the adult population of men and women over the age of 40. Prevention and treatment of glucocorticoid-induced OP encompasses variations in doses, durations, and patterns. Patients receiving higher doses of glucocorticoids (>30 mg/d) are at an increased risk and treatment plans should be tailored to those individual patients. In contrast with the published literature on postmenopausal OP, there is a paucity of data in the glucocorticoid-treated population.

Initial Evaluation

The history and physical of a patient treated with intermittent or long-term use of glucocorticoid medication is similar to that of the postmenopausal OP patient. After a thorough history of corticosteroid use is obtained, validated tools such as BMD, VFA, and FRAX should be used. The American College of Rheumatology 2017 Guidelines for Glucocorticoid Induced Osteoporosis recommend these tools be used early, and certainly no later 6 months after starting treatment. FRAX calculations assume a prednisone dose of 2.5 to 7.5 mg/d. The FRAX calculation should be adjusted upward for those patients on more than 7.5 mg/d by 15% for major osteoporotic fracture and by 20% for hip fracture.

Stratification of Risk

Indications for treatment for glucocorticoid-induced osteoporosis

All adults who are taking more than 2.5 mg/d of prednisone should optimize calcium intake (1000–1200 mgs daily) and vitamin D (600–800 IU daily), and optimize lifestyle changes reviewed in postmenopausal OP (**Table 2**).

Patients who are at low risk for fracture should optimize supplemental calcium and vitamin D intake over treatment with bisphosphonates and other OP medications. This recommendation is based on low-quality of evidence on additional fracture benefit of alternative treatments in this low-risk group.

Patients who are moderate risk and high risk for fracture should treat with an oral bisphosphonate in addition to calcium and vitamin D. If oral bisphosphonates are not tolerated or appropriate, the American College of Rheumatology guidelines recommend these treatments in this order: IV bisphosphonates, teriparatide, denosumab, and raloxifene.[60]

Table 2	
Fracture risk categories in glucocorticoid-treated patients	
Fracture Risk	**Adults >40 y**
Low	FRAX (glucocorticoid-adjusted[a]) 10-y risk of major osteoporotic fracture[b] <10% FRAX (glucocorticoid-adjusted[a]) 10-y risk of hip fracture ≤1%
Moderate	FRAX (glucocorticoid-adjusted[a]) 10-y risk of major osteoporotic fracture[b] 10%–19% FRAX (glucocorticoid-adjusted[a]) 10-y risk of hip fracture >1% and <3%
High	Prior osteoporotic fracture(s) BMD T-score of ≤−2.5 in the hip or spine In men age ≥50 and in postmenopausal women. FRAX (glucocorticoid adjusted[a]) 10 y risk of major osteoporotic fracture[b] ≥20% or (glucocorticoid adjusted[a]) 10-y risk of hip fracture ≥3%

[a] Increase the risk generated with N by 1.15 for major osteoporotic fracture and 1.2 for hip fracture if glucocorticoid treatment is 7.5 mg/d (eg, if hip fracture risk is 2.0%, increase to 2.4%).
[b] Major osteoporotic fracture includes fractures of the spine (clinical), hip, wrist, or humerus.
Adapted from Buckley L, Guyatt G, Fink HA, et al. 2017 American College of Rheumatology Guideline for the Prevention and Treatment of Glucocorticoid-Induced Osteoporosis [published correction appears in Arthritis Care Res (Hoboken). 2017 Nov;69(11):1776]. Arthritis Care Res (Hoboken). 2017;69(8):1095-1110. https://doi.org/10.1002/acr.23279; with permission.

Reassessment of Fracture Risk

The American College of Rheumatology 2017 guidelines recommend clinical risk factor reassessment for those 40 years of age and older and continuing glucocorticoid therapy to be followed every 1 to 3 years. Reassessment should be earlier for patients on OP medications, calcium and vitamin D if the initial prednisone dose was greater than 30 mg/d, and the cumulative dose is more than 5 g over the preceding year or those with a prior history of OP fracture(s). For those patients who have been on OP medications in the past and are no longer being treated with glucocorticoid, stopping the OP medication is recommended if the fracture risk is assessed to be low at the time of discontinuation. If the risk of fracture is high, then continuation of the medication is strongly recommended.[60]

Special Considerations: Male Osteoporosis

Definition and epidemiology

OP in men is an important entity. Although much of the discussion in this article regarding postmenopausal OP can apply, there are specific considerations for OP in men that must be considered. The epidemiologic statistics are alarming. OP affects an enormous number of people, including men of all ages and races. Among Caucasian adults in the United States aged 50 years and older, 20% of men will experience an osteoporotic fracture in their remaining lifetime.[62–64] An estimated 80,000 men fracture owing to OP annually in the United States.[65] Of these men, 30,000 die in the year after hip fracture, a fatality rate that is 50% higher than seen in women.[66] Morbidity is also higher in men after a fracture.[67]

Using a combination of lifestyle measures, and sometimes adding FDA-approved medications, OP and subsequent fractures can be prevented and treated. Unfortunately, underdiagnosis and treatment of men is an ongoing problem worldwide and it has been estimated that even among those who had sustained a hip fracture, fewer than 20% were assessed or treated.[68]

Sex-specific skeletal features in men

It is known that, in adolescence and early adulthood, androgens increase and estrogens decrease cortical bone size[69]; therefore, boys develop larger bones than girls and accrue a higher bone mass. This relative difference in bone size persists throughout life and provides resistance to fracture. Peak bone mass is reached between age 25 to 35 in males. Unlike women, men do not have a midlife loss of sex steroid production (menopause) and do not experience accelerated bone loss and an increase in fracture risk. In men, bone loss occurs slowly, starting at middle age. The Framingham Osteoporosis Study data showed that aging men (mean age, 75 years) lost about 1% of their bone mass annually.[70] **Fig. 5** compares bone loss in women and men over time.

Male risk factors for osteoporosis

There are several independent risk factors identified in large scale observational studies in men:[68]

- Advanced age
- Low body mass index
- Current smoking
- Excessive alcohol use
- Glucocorticoid use
- Personal history of fractures
- History of falls

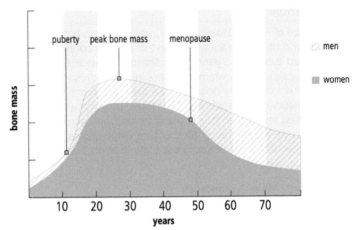

Fig. 5. Comparison of bone loss in women and men over time. (*From* Ebeling P. Osteoporosis in Men: Why Change Needs Happen. International Osteoporosis Foundation. Available at: http://share.iofbonehealth.org/WOD/2014/thematic-report/WOD14-Report.pdf.)

- Depression and use of antidepressants
- Hypogonadism
- History of stroke

A history of diabetes has also been noted to be an independent risk factor.[71–73] Additional risk factors are found in **Table 3**.

Table 3 Common risk factors for OP in men	
Medications	Glucocorticoid use of >7.5 mg/d for >3 mo
Nutritional	Low calcium Vitamin D insufficiency or deficiency
Gastrointratinal diseases and conditions	Malabsorption syndromes Gastrointratinal surgery Celiac disease
Hypogonadal States	Primary hypogonadism (defects of the testes), cryptorchidism, Klinefelter's syndrome XXY, glucocorticoids, alcohol Secondary hypogonadism (defects of the hypothalamus or pituitary gland) Functional: excessive exercise, weight change, low body mass index Structural: prolactinoma, cranial radiation, head trauma Iatrogenic: androgen deprivation therapy, opioids, marijuana, exogenous administration of androgens

From Ebeling P. Osteoporosis in Men: Why Change Needs Happen. International Osteoporosis Foundation. Available at: http://share.iofbonehealth.org/WOD/2014/thematic-report/WOD14-Report.pdf.

History

Taking a history for fracture in adulthood, height loss greater than 2.5 inches, a history of recent falls, a family history of OP, alcohol intake, smoking history, and medication history (especially corticosteroids) are all important. A history of delayed puberty, hypogonadism, prostate cancer (androgen deprivation therapy), hyperthyroidism, hyperparathyroidism, and chronic obstructive pulmonary disease are all important clues as to your patient's risk for fracture.

Physical Examination

Physical examination should pay close attention to height and weight measurement, observation of kyphosis, spinal tenderness on palpation, gait stability and fall risk evaluation, overall muscle tone, mobility, frailty, and respiratory examination for signs of chronic obstructive pulmonary disease. In men, a provider should look for testicular atrophy. An oral examination for those considering bisphosphonate therapy is always prudent.[68]

Laboratory Evaluation

The laboratory evaluation should include complete blood count, comprehensive metabolic panel, 25 (OH)D, and 24-hour urine calcium excretion. In men, also consider liver function tests and total testosterone. In the MrOS study of more than 1500 men aged 65 and older showed 2 laboratory values that were concerning regarding bone health. They were low vitamin D and alkaline phosphatase, both of which are linked to bone loss and can result from a multiplicity of pathologic processes associated with an increased risk for fracture.[74]

Indications for Treatment in Men

Men age 50 and older presenting with the following should be considered for treatment:

- T-score of −2.5 or less at the femoral neck, total hip, or lumbar spine
- A low trauma hip fracture (regardless of bone density)
- Fracture of vertebrae, proximal humerus, pelvis, or wrist in a setting of osteopenia (T-score between −1.0 and −2.5)
- Low bone mass (T-score between −1.0 and −2.5 at the femoral neck or lumbar spine) and a 10-year probability of a hip fracture of 3% or higher or a 10-year probability of a major OP-related fracture of 20% or higher based on the US-adapted WHO algorithm[9]

UNIVERSAL RECOMMENDATIONS

Men at risk for OP should be counseled on the same universal recommendations as for postmenopausal OP. In particular, men should be educated on avoiding excess alcohol intake, smoking cessation, and adequate dietary intake of calcium and vitamin D.

PHARMACOLOGIC MANAGEMENT

As with postmenopausal OP, selection of medication in men is determined by the individual and their preference. The FDA has approved bisphosphonates (alendronate, risedronate, and zoledronic acid), teriparatide, and denosumab. All FDA-approved medications have shown efficacy in randomized controlled trials to increase BMD. Data for fracture reduction exist, but are more limited. In a meta-analysis of 22 studies, fewer vertebral fractures were demonstrated in men taking alendronate with a 69% reduction and risedronate showing a 57% reduction, but no vertebral fracture reduction in men taking calcitonin or denosumab.[75] The US Preventive Services Task Force in a different meta-analysis with zoledronic acid showed a decrease in of morphometric vertebral fractures in men of 67% with no decrease in clinical vertebral fractures or hip fracture.[76] In men with prostate cancer being treated with androgen deprivation therapy, denosumab showed a significant decrease in new vertebral fractures in men treated for 3 years compared with placebo of 1.5% versus 3.9%.[77]

Men who have serum testosterone levels of less than 200 ng/mL on more than 1 determination and who have signs and symptoms of androgen deficiency should be considered for testosterone therapy. Additionally, if there is evidence of high risk for OP, FDA-approved OP medications should be recommended.

Monitoring

The National Osteoporosis Foundation, Endocrine Society, and American Association of Clinical Endocrinologists/American College of Endocrinology recommend annual follow-up, which should include a history of fracture(s), new falls, new or worsening comorbidities, and medication reconciliation. Height loss of more than 0.8 inches since the last office visit and new or worsening back pain should be evaluated with radiograph or VFA.[78] Repeat BMD should be performed every 2 years or earlier if new fractures or unexpected medical history warrants, but less frequently if an upward or stable trend has been documented.

SUMMARY

More than 50 million people in the United States are estimated to either have OP or low bone mass. OP is a major public health threat as 2 million fractures occur annually as a result of this disease. One in 2 women will fracture a bone in their lifetime and this incidence is greater than the combined occurrences of myocardial infarction, stroke, and breast cancer. In the United States, men over the age of 50 also suffer from OP. In the United States, 80,000 men fracture annually owing to OP and of those 30,000 will die after a hip fracture, more than twice the fatality rate seen in women.

Fractures can be prevented by recognizing the multiple risk factors, including coexisting disease states and medications that are deleterious to bone. The use of validated tools such as BMD, DXA scanning, the FRAX tool, TBS, VFA, and bone turnover markers have added to our tools for measuring bone density and bone quality.

Since 1995, with the release of alendronate, the understanding of bone metabolism has been greatly enhanced. Presently, there are several categories of effective medications that treat and prevent fractures with very acceptable side effect profiles. Primary care physicians, PAs, and NPs are on the front line for evaluation, diagnosis, and management of OP. Understanding the broad strokes of bone health and risk for fracture are important if we are to make a difference in our patient's lives and reverse the trend of under-recognition and undertreatment.

CLINICS CARE POINTS

Indications for treatment include the following:
- T-score of −2.5 or less at the femoral neck, total hip, or lumbar spine
- A low trauma hip fracture (regardless of bone density)

- Fracture of vertebrae, proximal humerus, pelvis, or wrist in a setting of osteopenia (T-score between −1.0 and −2.5) and a 10-year probability of a hip fracture of 3% or higher or a 10-year probability of a major OP-related fracture of 20% or higher based on the US-adapted WHO algorithm
- DXA scans are recommended for all women 65 and older
- DXA scans are recommended for all men age 70 and older
- The FRAX calculator can estimate fracture risk going forward 10 years and can be found on the Internet at: https://www.sheffield.ac.uk/FRAX/
- Universal recommendations include regular calcium in diet and supplements, vitamin D supplements, regular weight-bearing exercise, balance training, muscle strengthening, well-rounded nutritional intake, discontinuing smoking, limiting alcohol intake, and evaluation of patients for fall risk

DISCLOSURE

Authors have nothing to disclose.

REFERENCES

1. Burge R, Dawson-Hughes B, Solomon DH, et al. Incidence and economic burden of osteoporosis-related fractures in the US, 2005-2025. J Bone Miner Res 2007; 22(3):465–75.
2. Morin SN, Lix LM, Leslie WD. The importance of previous fracture sites on osteoporosis diagnosis and incident fractures in women. J Bone Miner Res 2014;29: 1695.
3. Kanis JA, De Laet C, Delmas P, et al. A meta-analysis of previous fracture and fracture risk. Bone 2004;35:375–82.
4. Margolis KL, Ensrud KE, Schreiner PJ, et al. Body size and risk for clinical fractures in older women. Study of Osteoporotic Fractures Research Group. Ann Intern Med 2000;133(2):123–7.
5. Siminoski K, Jiang G, Adachi JD, et al. Accuracy of height loss during prospective monitoring for detection of incident vertebral fractures. Osteoporos Int 2005; 16:403–10.
6. Tannenbaum C, Clark J, Schwartzman K, et al. Yield of Laboratory Testing to Identify Secondary Contributors to Osteoporosis in Otherwise Healthy Women. J Clin Endocrinol Metab 2002;87(10):4431–43.
7. International Society for Clinical Densitometry. 2015 ISCD adult official positions.2015. Available at: https://www.iscd.org/official-positions/2019-iscd-official-positions-adult/
8. Kanis JA, Harvey NC, Cooper C, et al, Advisory Board of the National Osteoporosis Guideline Group. A systematic review of intervention thresholds based on FRAX: a report prepared for the National Osteoporosis Guideline Group and the International Osteoporosis Foundation. Arch Osteoporos 2016;11(1):25.
9. Siris ES, Adler R, Bilzekian J, et al. The clinical diagnosis of Osteoporosis. A position statement from the Nation Bone Health Alliance Working Group. Osteoporos Int 2014;25:1439–43.
10. Cosman F, de Beur SJ, LeBoff MS, et al. Clinician's guide to prevention and treatment of osteoporosis. Osteoporos Int 2014;25(10):2359–81.
11. Prentice RL, Pettinger MB, Jackson RD, et al. Health risks and benefits from calcium and vitamin D supplementation: Women's Health Initiative clinical trial and cohort study. Osteoporos Int 2013;24(2):567–80.

12. Bolland MJ, Grey A, Avenell A, et al. Calcium supplements with or without vitamin D and risk of cardiovascular events: reanalysis of the Women's Health Initiative limited access dataset and meta-analysis. BMJ 2011;19:342.

13. Silverman SL, Cummings SR, Watts NB. Consensus Panel of the ASBMR, ISCD, and NOF. Recommendations for the clinical evaluation of agents for treatment of osteoporosis: consensus of an expert panel representing the American Society for Bone and Mineral Research (ASBMR), the International Society for Clinical Densitometry (ISCD), and the National Osteoporosis Foundation (NOF). J Bone Miner Res 2008;23:159–65.

14. Chapuy MC, Preziosi P, Maamer M, et al. Prevalence of vitamin D insufficiency in an adult normal population. Osteoporos Int 1997;7:439–43.

15. Dawson-Hughes B, Heaney RP, Holick MF, et al. Estimates of optimal vitamin D status. Osteoporos Int 2005;16:713–6.

16. Bischoff-Ferrari HA, Giovannucci E, Willett WC, et al. Estimation of optimal serum concentrations of 25-hydroxyvitamin D for multiple health outcomes. Am J Clin Nutr 2006;84(1):18–28.

17. DIPART (Vitamin D Individual Patient Analysis of Randomized Trials) Group. Patient level pooled analysis of 68 500 patients from seven major vitamin D fracture trials in US and Europe. BMJ 2010;340:b5463.

18. Robertson MC, Ampbell AJ, Gardner MM, et al. Preventing injuries in older people by preventing falls: a meta-analysis of individual-level data. J Am Geriatr Soc 2002;50(5):905–11.

19. Kelley GA, Kelley KS, Kohrt WM. Effects of ground and joint reaction force exercise on lumbar spine and femoral neck bone mineral density in postmenopausal women: a meta-analysis of randomized controlled trials. BMC Musculoskelet Disord 2012;13:177.

20. Krall EA, Dawson-Hughes B. Smoking and bone loss among postmenopausal women. J Bone Mineral Res 1991;6(4):331–8.

21. Law MR, Hackshaw AK. A meta-analysis of cigarette smoking, bone mineral density and risk of hip fracture: recognition of a major effect. BMJ 1997;315(7112): 841–6.

22. Kanis JA, Johansson H, Johnell O, et al. Alcohol intake as a risk factor for fracture. Osteoporos Int 2005;16(7):737–42.

23. Cummings SR, Joseph Melton L. Epidemiology and outcomes of osteoporotic fractures. Lancet 2002;359(9319):1761–7.

24. Cumming RG, Salkeld G, Thomas M, et al. Prospective Study of the Impact of Fear of Falling on Activities of Daily Living, SF-36 Scores, and Nursing Home Admission. J Gerontol A Biol Sci Med Sci 2000;55(5):M299–305.

25. Eastel RI, Rosen CJ, Black DM, et al. Pharmacological management of osteoporosis in postmenopausal women: an Endocrine Society Clinical Practice Guideline. J Clin Endocrinol Metab 2019;104(5):1595–622.

26. Anderson G, Limacher M, Assaf A, et al. Effects of conjugated equine estrogen in postmenopausal women with hysterectomy: the Women's Health Initiative randomized controlled trial. JAMA 2004;291(14):1701–12.

27. Cauley JA, Norton L, Lippman ME, et al. Continued breast cancer risk reduction in postmenopausal women treated with raloxifene: 4-year results from the MORE trial. Multiple outcomes of raloxifene evaluation. Breast Cancer Res Treat 2001; 65(2):125–34.

28. Martino S, Cauley JA, Barrett-Connor E, et al. CORE Investigators. Continuing outcomes relevant to Evista: breast cancer incidence in postmenopausal

osteoporotic women in a randomized trial of raloxifene. J Natl Cancer Inst 2004; 96(23):1751–61.

29. Vogel VG, Costantino JP, Wickerham DL, et al. National Surgical Adjuvant Breast and Bowel Project (NSABP). Effects of tamoxifen vs. raloxifene on the risk of developing invasive breast cancer and other disease outcomes: the NSABP Study of Tamoxifen and Raloxifene (STAR) P-2 trial. JAMA 2006;295(23):2727–41.

30. Barrett-Connor E, Mosca L, Collins P, et al. Raloxifene Use for The Heart (RUTH) Trial Investigators. Effects of raloxifene on cardiovascular events and breast cancer in postmenopausal women. N Engl J Med 2006;355(2):125–37.

31. Harris ST, Watts NB, Genant HK, et al. Effects of risedronate treatment on vertebral and nonvertebral fractures in women with postmenopausal osteoporosis: a randomized controlled trial. Vertebral Efficacy With Risedronate Therapy (VERT) Study Group. JAMA 1999;282:1344–52.

32. Reginster J, Minne HW, Sorensen OH, et al. Randomized trial of the effects of risedronate on vertebral fractures in women with establish postmenopausal osteoporosis. Efficacy of Risedronate Therapy (VERT) Study Group. Osteoporos Int 2000;11:83–91.

33. Black DM, Delmas PD, Eastell R, et al. Once yearly zoledronic acid for treatment of postmenopausal osteoporosis. N Engl J Med 2007;356:1809–22.

34. Cummings SR, Black DM, Thompson DE, et al. Effect of alendronate on risk of fracture in women with low bone density but without vertebral fractures: results from the Fracture Intervention Trial. JAMA 1998;280:2077–82.

35. Camacho PM, Petak SM, Binkley N, et al, American Association of Clinical Endocrinologists. Clinical Practice Guidelines for the diagnosis and treatment of postmenopausal osteoporosis. Endocr Pract 2016;22(Suppl 4).

36. Fosamax *TM* prescribing information. Drugs@FDA: FDA approved drug products: Updated 2012. Available at: https://www.accessdata.fda.gov/drugsatfda_docs/label/2004/20560slr030,21575slr002_fosamax_lbl.pdf.

37. Rosen H. The use of bisphosphonates in postmenopausal women with osteoporosis. UpToDate; 2019.

38. Kidney Disease: Improving Global Outcomes KDIGO CKD-MBD Work Group. KDIGO clinical practice guideline for the diagnosis, evaluation, prevention, and treatment of Chronic Kidney Disease-Mineral and Bone Disorder (CKD-MBD). Kidney Int Suppl 2009;(113):S1–130.

39. Black DM, Reid IR, Boonen S, et al. The effect of 3 versus 6 years of Zoledronic acid treatment of osteoporosis: a randomized extension to the HORIZON-Pivotal Fracture Trial. J Bone Miner Res 2012;27(2):243–54.

40. Lyles KW, Colón-Emeric CS, Magaziner JS, et al. Zoledronic acid and clinical fractures and mortality after hip fracture. N Engl J Med 2007;357(18):1799–809.

41. Highlights of Prescribing information- Reclast Injection Initial US approval 2001. Available at: https://www.pharma.us.novartis.com/sites/www.pharma.us.novartis.com/files/reclast.pdf. Accessed February 22, 2020.

42. Cummings SR, San Martin J, McClung MR, et al. FREEDOM Trial. Denosumab for prevention of fractures in postmenopausal women with osteoporosis. N Engl J Med 2009;361(8):756–65. Erratum appears in N Engl J Med. 2009;361(19):1914].

43. Zaheer S, LeBoff M, Lewiecki EM. Denosumab for the treatment of osteoporosis. Expert Opin Drug Metab Toxicol 2015;11(3):461–70.

44. Cummings SR, Ferrari S, Eastell R, et al. Vertebral fractures after discontinuation of denosumab: a post hoc analysis of the randomized placebo-controlled FREEDOM Trial and its extension. J Bone Miner Res 2018;33:190–8.

45. Tsourdi E, Langdahl B, Cohen-Solal M, et al. A discontinuation of denosumab therapy for osteoporosis: a systematic review position statement by ECTS. Bone 2017;105:11–7.

46. Silverman SL, Zaidi M, Lewiecki EM, et al. Postmenopausal Osteoporosis: putting the risk for osteonecrosis of the jaw into perspective. Medscape Online CME.

47. Hellstein JW, Adler RA, Edwards B, et al. Managing the care of patients receiving antiresorptive therapy for prevention and treatment of osteoporosis: Executive Summary of the Recommendations from the American Dental Association Council on Scientific Affairs. J Am Dent Assoc 2011;142(11):1243–55.

48. Shane E, Burr D, Abrahamsen B, et al. Atypical subtrochanteric and diaphyseal femoral fractures: second report of a task force of the American Society for Bone and Mineral Research. J Bone Miner Res 2014;29:1–23.

49. Neer RM, Arnaud CD, Zanchetta JR, et al. Effect of parathyroid hormone (1–34) on fractures and bone mineral density in postmenopausal women with osteoporosis. N Engl J Med 2001;344:1434–41.

50. Miller PD, Hattersley G, Riis BJ, et al. ACTIVE Study Investigators. Effect of abaloparatide vs placebo on new vertebral fractures in postmenopausal women with osteoporosis: a randomized clinical trial. JAMA 2016;316(7):722–33.

51. Cosman F, Miller PD, Williams GC, et al. Eighteen months of treatment with subcutaneous abaloparatide followed by 6 months of treatment with alendronate in postmenopausal women with osteoporosis: results of the ACTIVExtend Trial. Mayo Clin Proc 2017;92(2):200–10.

52. Haas AV, LeBoff MS. Osteoanabolic Agents for Osteoporosis. J Endocr Soc 2018; 2(8):922–32.

53. Package insert Forteo. Available at: https://pi.lilly.com/us/forteo-pi.pdf. Accessed February 15, 2020.

54. Keaveny TM, Crittenden DB, Bolognese MA, et al. Greater gains in spine and hip strength for romosozumab compared with teriparatide in postmenopausal women with low bone mass. J Bone Miner Res 2017;32(9):1956–62.

55. Genant HK, Engelke K, Bolognese MA, et al. Effects of romosozumab compared with teriparatide on bone density and mass at the spine and hip in postmenopausal women with low bone mass. J Bone Miner Res 2017;32(1):181–7.

56. Cosman F, Crittenden DB, Ferrari S, et al. Romosozumab FRAME Study: a post hoc analysis of the role of regional background fracture risk on nonvertebral fracture outcome. J Bone Miner Res 2018;33(8):1407–16.

57. McClung MR, Brown JP, Diez-Perez A, et al. Effects of 24 months of treatment with romosozumab followed by 12 months of denosumab or placebo in postmenopausal women with low bone mineral density: a randomized, double-blind, phase 2, parallel group study. J Bone Miner Res 2018;33(8):1397–406.

58. www.evenityhcp.com/ Product Insert EVENITY ® official site for physicians. Available at: https://www.pi.amgen.com/~/media/amgen/repositorysites/pi-amgen-com/evenity/evenity_pi.ashx. Accessed February 23, 2010.

59. Miller AN, Lake AF, Emory CL. Establishing a fracture liaison service: an orthopedic approach. J Bone Joint Surg Am 2015;97(8):675–81.

60. Buckley L, Guyatt G, Fink HA. 2017 American College of Rheumatology Guideline for the Prevention and Treatment of Glucocorticoid-Induced Osteoporosis. Arthritis Rheumatol 2017;69(8):1521–37.

61. Allen CS, Yeung JH. Bisphosphonates for steroid-induced osteoporosis. Cochrane Database Syst Rev 2016;(10):CD001347.

62. Melton LJ 3rd, Atkinson EJ, O'Connor MK, et al. Bone density and fracture risk in men. J Bone Miner Res 1998;13:191563.

63. Melton LJ 3rd, Chrischilles EA, Cooper C, et al. Perspective. How many women have osteoporosis? J Bone Miner Res 1992;7:1005.

64. Kanis JA, Johnell O, Oden A, et al. Long-term risk of osteoporotic fracture in Malmo. Osteoporos Int 2000;11:669.

65. Forsen I, Sogaard AJ, Meyer HE, et al. survival after hip fracture: short and long term excess mortality according to age and gender. Osteoporos Int 1999; 101(1):73–8.

66. Bentler SE, Liu L, Obrizan M, et al. The aftermath of hip fracture: discharge placement, functional status change and mortality. Am J Epidemiol 2009;170(10): 1290–9.

67. Bass E, French DD, Bradhan DD, et al. Risk adjusted mortality rates of elderly veterans with hip fractures. Ann Epidemiol 2007;17(7):514–9.

68. Ebeling PR. Osteoporosis in Men. Why Change Needs to Happen. N Engl J Med 2014;358:1474–82.

69. Lorentzon M, Swanson C, Andersson N, et al. Free testosterone is a positive, whereas free estradiol is a negative, predictor of cortical bone size in young Swedish men. J Bone Miner Res 2005;20:1334–41.

70. Hannan MT, Felson DT, Dawson-Hughes B. Risk factors for longitudinal bone loss in elderly men and women. The Framingham Osteoporosis Study. J Bone Miner Res 2000;15(4):710–20.

71. Lewis CE, Ewing SK, Taylor BC, et al. Osteoporotic Fractures in Men (MrOS) Study Research Group, authors. Predictors of non-spine fracture in elderly men: The MrOS study. J Bone Miner Res 2007;22(2):211–9.

72. Drake MT, Murad MD, Mauck KF, et al. authors. Clinical review. Risk factors for low bone mass-related fractures in men: a systematic review and meta-analysis. J Clin Endocrinol Metab 2012;97(6):1861–70.

73. Felson DT, Kile DP, Anderson JJ, et al. Alcohol consumption and hip fractures: the Framingham Study. Am J Epidemiol 1988;128(5):1102–10.

74. Fink HA, Litwack-Harrison S, Taylor BC, et al. Clinical utility of routine laboratory testing to identify possible secondary causes in older men with osteoporosis: the Osteoporotic Fractures in Men (MrOS) Study. Osteoporos Int 2016;27:331–8.

75. Nayak S, Greenspan SL. Osteoporosis treatment efficacy for men: a systematic review and meta-analysis. J Am Geriatr Soc 2017;65(3):490–5.

76. Viswanathan M, Reddy S, Berkman N, et al. Screening to prevent osteoporotic fractures: updated evidence report and systematic review for the US Preventive Services Task Force. JAMA 2018;319(24):2532–51.

77. Lipton A, Smith MR, Ellis GK, et al. Treatment-induced bone loss and fractures in cancer patients undergoing hormone ablation therapy: efficacy and safety of denosumab. Clin Med Insights Oncol 2012;6:287–303.

78. Hillier TA, Lui LY, Kado DM, et al. Height loss in older women: risk of hip fracture and mortality independent of vertebral fractures. J Bone Miner Res 2012;27(1): 153–9.

Axial Spondyloarthritis and Ankylosing Spondylitis

Anand Kumthekar, MBBS[a],*, Atul Deodhar, MD, FRCP[b]

KEYWORDS

- Axial spondyloarthritis • Ankylosing spondylitis
- Nonradiographic axial spondyloarthritis • Radiographic axial spondyloarthritis

KEY POINTS

- Axial spondyloarthritis (axSpA) is an umbrella term that includes ankylosing spondylitis (AS) and nonradiographic axSpA (nr-axSpA).
- HLA-B27 test is not essential for a diagnosis of axSpA. Rather, the diagnosis of axSpA should be based on clinical features of chronic low back pain (usually inflammatory) starting before the age of 45, plus extra-articular manifestations of spondyloarthritis (eg, psoriasis, peripheral arthritis, iritis, inflammatory bowel disease, enthesitis) with imaging evidence of sacroiliitis (radiograph and/or MRI).
- A single Ferguson view of the pelvis is optimal for diagnosis of sacroiliitis. When radiograph is normal or equivocal, MRI of the sacroiliac joints (without contrast) should be ordered to detect active inflammation.
- Treatment goals of axSpA include reducing pain, stiffness, and fatigue, along with prevention of disease progression and structural damage, leading to reduced disability, and improving health-related quality of life. Physical therapy is an important aspect of treatment along with drug therapy, such as nonsteroidal anti-inflammatory drugs, TNF-inhibitors, and IL-17A inhibitors.

INTRODUCTION

Spondyloarthritis (SpA) is a group of chronic inflammatory diseases characterized by common clinical, genetic, and etiopathogenic features. It includes axial SpA (axSpA) and peripheral SpA, such as psoriatic arthritis, reactive arthritis, and enteropathic arthritis. The axial skeleton including the spine and sacroiliac joints are predominantly affected in axSpA. axSpA is an umbrella term that includes ankylosing spondylitis (AS; also called radiographic axSpA) and nonradiographic axSpA (nr-axSpA) (**Fig. 1**). The hallmark feature of AS is definitive evidence of radiographic sacroiliitis, whereas in nr-axSpA there is no definitive radiographic sacroiliitis but MRI can show evidence

[a] Montefiore Medical Center, Albert Einstein College of Medicine, 1250 Waters Place, Tower II, 12th Floor, Bronx, NY 10461, USA; [b] Oregon Health & Science University, 3181 Southwest Sam Jackson Park Road, Portland 97239, USA
* Corresponding author.
E-mail addresses: Anand.kumthekar@gmail.com; anakumth@montefiore.org

Physician Assist Clin 6 (2021) 135–147
https://doi.org/10.1016/j.cpha.2020.09.005
2405-7991/21/© 2020 Elsevier Inc. All rights reserved.
physicianassistant.theclinics.com

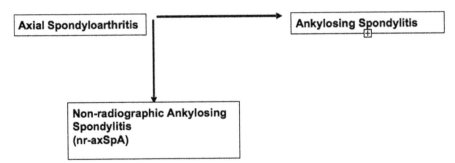

Fig. 1. Classification of axial spondyloarthritis.

of sacroiliitis. It is now accepted that nr-axSpA and AS are a continued spectrum of the same disease process **(Fig. 2)**.[1]

HOW COMMON IS AXIAL SPONDYLOARTHRITIS?

axSpA usually presents in the second or third decade of life, and rarely in patients with onset of back pain after the age of 45 years. It has been closely associated with HLA-B27. Its prevalence runs in parallel with HLA-B27 distribution among different races and thus is higher in White populations compared with African Americans. In the general population, axSpA is likely to develop in approximately 5% of the HLA-B27-positive individuals, whereas that risk increases to 10% to 30% if they have a first-degree relative with HLA-B27-positive AS.[2,3] The prevalence of axSpA in the United States from the 2009 to 2010 US National Health and Nutrition Examination Survey is estimated to be 0.9% to 1.4% based on the Amor and European Spondylarthropathy Study Group criteria, respectively.[4]

WHAT ARE THE REASONS FOR LATE DIAGNOSIS OF AXIAL SPONDYLOARTHRITIS?

Back pain is common in the general population and affects approximately 80% of all adults at some point in their life time. The diagnosis of axSpA can be delayed by 8 to

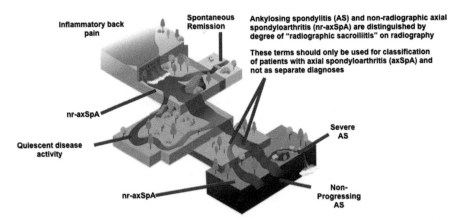

Fig. 2. Concept of axSpA illustrating nr-axSpA and axSpA as a continued spectrum of the same disease. (*Adapted from* van Vollenhoven RF. Unresolved issues in biologic therapy for rheumatoid arthritis. Nat Rev Rheumatol. 2011;7(4):205-215. https://doi.org/10.1038/nrrheum.2011.22; with permission.)

10 years after first symptom onset.[5] Chronic lower back pain affects 13% of adults between 20 and 69 years of age[6] and inflammatory back pain (IBP) accounts for only 5% to 6% of all chronic back pain.[7] One of the most obvious reasons for the long diagnostic delay is the high burden of mechanical back pain in the general population. Another obvious reason is that there is no validated diagnostic criteria for the diagnosis of axSpA.[8] The modified New York criteria (**Box 1**) for classification of AS[9] requires the presence of radiographic sacroiliitis. It is widely used in clinical practice for making diagnosis, even though it is known that radiographic sacroiliitis can take many years after the onset of symptoms to be visible on plain radiographs. Thus, sensitivity of modified New York criteria for diagnosis of axSpA is poor.

CLASSIFICATION CRITERIA

The Assessment of SpondyloArthritis International Society (ASAS) published new classification criteria for axSpA (**Fig. 3**).[10,11] The ASAS group proposed that a patient could be classified as having axSpA by fulfilling one of two arms after satisfying the entry criteria of onset of back pain before 45 years and having more than 3 months of chronic back pain. The clinical arm allowed classification based on a positive HLA-B27 test and two or more SpA features. These features include IBP, peripheral inflammatory arthritis, heel enthesitis, uveitis, dactylitis, psoriasis, inflammatory bowel disease (ie, Crohn disease and ulcerative colitis), good response to nonsteroidal anti-inflammatory drugs (NSAIDs), family history of SpA, or an elevated C-reactive protein (CRP). The imaging arm allowed classification based on either a positive MRI or radiographic sacroiliitis and one or more SpA features. These criteria were developed for research purposes and not to make a clinical diagnosis.

WHY IS EARLY DIAGNOSIS IMPORTANT?

The diagnosis of axSpA is challenging because of higher prevalence of back pain in the population but an early diagnosis has important implications. Clinical manifestations and disease activity measures are highly comparable between patients with nr-axSpA and AS.[12] A good functional status along with a short disease duration has shown to predict a good response to tumor necrosis factor inhibitor (TNFi) therapy.[13] Early diagnosis of axSpA is associated with better outcomes in disease activity, function, spinal mobility, and/or radiographic damage.[14,15] Patients with a shorter

---

Box 1
Modified New York criteria for ankylosing spondylitis

1. Clinical criteria
   a. Low back pain and stiffness for more than 3 months, which improves with rest but not with exercise.
   b. Limitation of motion of the lumbar spine in sagittal and frontal planes.
   c. Limitation of chest expansion relative to normal values for age and sex.

2. Radiologic criterion
   Sacroiliitis grade 2 bilaterally or sacroiliitis grade 3 to 4 unilaterally.

Definite ankylosing spondylitis is present if the radiologic criterion is associated with at least one clinical criteria.

Data from van der Linden S, Valkenburg HA, Cats A. Evaluation of diagnostic criteria for ankylosing spondylitis. A proposal for modification of the New York criteria. *Arthritis Rheum.* 1984;27(4):361-368. https://doi.org/10.1002/art.1780270401.

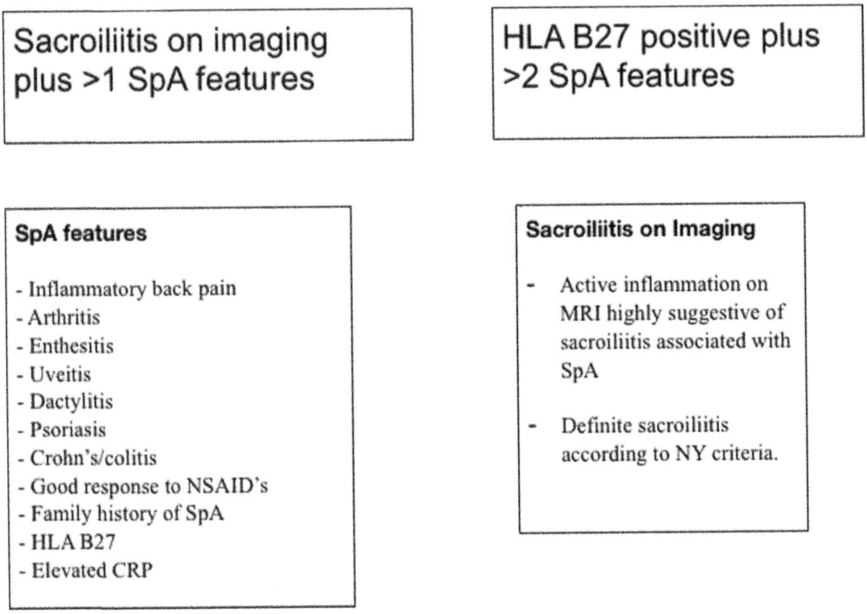

Sacroiliitis on imaging plus >1 SpA features	HLA B27 positive plus >2 SpA features

SpA features

- Inflammatory back pain
- Arthritis
- Enthesitis
- Uveitis
- Dactylitis
- Psoriasis
- Crohn's/colitis
- Good response to NSAID's
- Family history of SpA
- HLA B27
- Elevated CRP

Sacroiliitis on Imaging

- Active inflammation on MRI highly suggestive of sacroiliitis associated with SpA

- Definite sacroiliitis according to NY criteria.

Fig. 3. ASAS classification criteria for axSpA. CRP, C-reactive protein; NSAID, nonsteroidal anti-inflammatory drug. (*From* Rudwaleit M, van der Heijde D, Landewe R, et al. The development of Assessment of Spondy-loArthritis international Society classification criteria for axial spondyloarthritis (part II): vali-dation and final selection. Ann Rheum Dis. 2009;68(6):777-78; with permission.)

disease duration are more likely to respond to biologic agents than were patients with long-standing disease.[16] Thus, having a high suspicion of axSpA in the right clinical context and ordering appropriate imaging studies helps in the early diagnosis of axSpA.

CLUES FOR EARLY DIAGNOSIS/CLINICAL FEATURES
Articular Manifestations

Low back pain
Back pain is a cardinal feature of axSpA and because back pain is so prevalent in the population, it is important to note that back pain caused by axSpA is usually different from mechanical back pain. According to ASAS criteria a patient has IBP if four out of the five parameters are present (**Box 2**).[17] Back pain in axSpA is mostly inflammatory in nature that is often associated with morning stiffness, improves with physical activity, is better by midday, and not relieved by rest. It is relieved by the use of NSAIDs. Buttock pain is an important distinguishing feature of IBP and it typically alternates from side to side. Patients may complain of back pain that is worse in the second half of night that can cause poor sleep. Fatigue as a result of chronic back pain and stiffness may be an important problem and is accentuated by sleep disturbances caused by these symptoms.

Peripheral joint pain
Inflammatory arthritis, which is usually asymmetric, oligoarticular (one to four joints), and involving the lower extremities is seen in patients with axSpA (**Fig. 4**). Dactylitis

> **Box 2**
> **ASAS criteria for IBP**
>
> IBP according to ASAS, which is to be applied in patients with chronic back pain for <3 months
> Age at onset <40 years
> Insidious onset
> Improvement with exercise
> No improvement with rest
> Pain at night (with improvement on getting up)
>
> Need at least four out of five parameters to classify as IBP.
>
> *Data from* Sieper, J., Rudwaleit, M., Baraliakos, X et al. The Assessment of SpondyloArthritis International Society (ASAS) handbook: a guide to assess spondyloarthritis. Ann Rheum Dis 2009, 68(Suppl 2), ii1-ii44.

or sausage digit is inflammation of the entire finger or toe, and is rarely seen in axSpA (**Fig. 5**).

Enthesitis
Enthesitis is defined as inflammation at the insertion of muscles, ligaments, or tendons on bones, at such sites as the Achilles tendon. Tenderness on palpation at the site of entheseal insertion is a central feature of axSpA (**Fig. 6**). Tenderness on palpation of the costosternal junctions, greater trochanters, tibial tubercles, and heels (Achilles tendinitis or plantar fasciitis) is also seen in axSpA. Patients can have chest pain caused by enthesitis at the costosternal and manubriosternal joint, which is worse with coughing or sneezing.

Extraskeletal Manifestations

Uveitis
Uveitis associated with axSpA is acute anterior uveitis, which is usually sudden, recurrent, and unilateral (**Fig. 7**). Patients with axSpA are at a higher risk of uveitis and it is estimated that uveitis can occur in 50% of patients with axSpA.[18] A patient with acute anterior uveitis and HLA-B27-positive is at a higher risk of developing axSpA.[19]

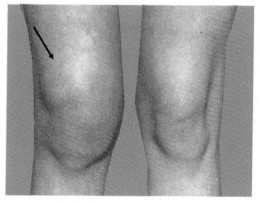

Fig. 4. Acute inflammatory arthritis. (*From* ASAS slide kit. Available at: www.asas-group. org/.)

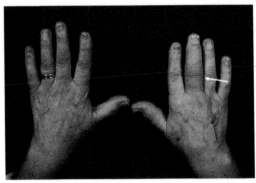

Fig. 5. Dactylitis of the right middle finger in a patient with psoriasis. * Psoriasis (*From* ASAS slide kit. Available at: www.asas-group.org/.)

Skin manifestations

Psoriasis is the most common skin manifestation of SpA (**Fig. 8**).[20] Patients with psoriasis can have articular symptoms in the form of oligoarticular peripheral inflammatory arthritis. Axial skeletal involvement is usually unilateral sacroiliitis and nonmarginal thick syndesmophyte formation. Other skin lesions associated with axSpA are circinate balanitis and keratoderma blennorrhagicum.

LABORATORY TESTING

There are no laboratory tests that can help confirm or exclude a diagnosis of axSpA. Elevated levels of CRP in the right clinical context can provide an additional clue to the clinician to make a diagnosis. Erythrocyte sedimentation rate is less useful than CRP in axSpA. Although HLA-B27 does not make the diagnosis of axSpA, its presence increases the likelihood of the diagnosis in the right context.

IMAGING
Radiograph Sacroiliac Joint

Imaging of the sacroiliac joint is crucial for correct and early diagnosis of axSpA (**Fig. 9**).[17] Conventional radiograph of the sacroiliac joints is recommended as the first

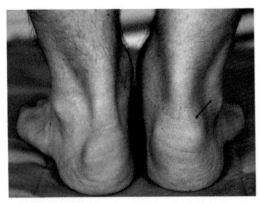

Fig. 6. Enthesitis of the right Achilles tendon. (*From* ASAS slide kit. Available at: www.asas-group.org/.)

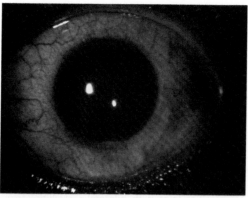

Fig. 7. Acute anterior uveitis in a patient with HLA-B27-positive ankylosing spondylitis. (*Courtesy of* C. Castiblanco, MD.)

imaging modality to diagnose sacroiliitis.[9,21,22] A single Ferguson view of the pelvis is ideal to diagnose sacroiliitis. Radiographic changes in the sacroiliac joints vary depending on the duration of disease because structural changes take months to years to take place.[23] Radiographic changes include subchondral sclerosis, uniform joint space narrowing, erosions, and finally ankylosis. Limitation of sacroiliac radiographs include the challenging interpretation even for an experienced radiologist and a substantial interreader variability.[24,25]

MRI Sacroiliac Joint

MRI should be obtained if the results of the sacroiliac joint radiograph are normal or equivocal and there is clinical suspicion for axSpA (**Fig. 10**).[22] The T2-weighted

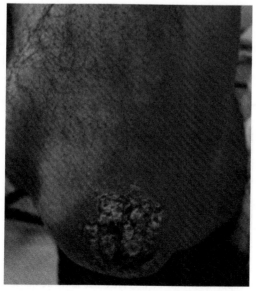

Fig. 8. Skin psoriasis. (*Courtesy of* L. Bizzocchi, MD and B. Ayesha, MD.)

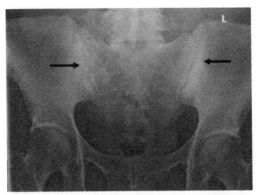

Fig. 9. Radiograph of sacroiliac joint with bilateral sacroiliitis (*arrows*). (*Courtesy of* A. Kumethekar.)

sequence with fat suppression (also called STIR image) is useful to detect active inflammatory changes, such as bone marrow edema (see **Fig. 10**).[26] A T1-weighted sequence helps to detect postinflammatory changes, such as erosions, sclerosis, and ankylosis. Contrast is not required for diagnosis of axSpA.

Spine

Spinal disease in axSpA is characterized by syndesmophyte formation (**Fig. 11**).[26] Syndesmophytes are thin, vertical bony projections that develop from ossification of the outer fibers of the annulus fibrosus of the intervertebral disk. They are visible on the anterior and lateral aspects of the spine and can bridge the intervertebral disk, causing ankylosis. Extensive syndesmophyte formation seen in advanced axSpA produces the classical bamboo spine.

MANAGEMENT

The treatment goals of axSpA are reducing pain, discomfort, and disability and preventing disease progression and structural damage. It includes physical therapy and pharmacotherapy including NSAIDs, TNFi, and interleukin-17 (IL-17A) inhibitors, which have been included in the latest American College of Rheumatology (ACR)/

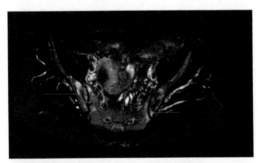

Fig. 10. Axial T2 fat-suppressed MRI of the sacroiliac joint demonstrating bone marrow edema (*arrows*). (*Courtesy of* A. Kumethekar.)

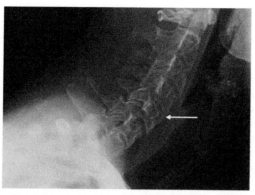

Fig. 11. Radiograph of the cervical spine showing thin syndesmophyte formation (*arrow*) in advanced ankylosing spondylitis.

Spondylitis Association of America (SAA)/Spondyloarthritis Research and Treatment Network (SPARTAN) guidelines (**Fig. 12**).[27]

Physical Therapy

Physical therapy is an important aspect of nonpharmacologic treatment of axSpA. The 2019 ACR/SAA/SPARTAN treatment guidelines recommend treatment with physical therapy over no treatment with physical therapy. It is also further recommended to have active and land-based physical therapy over passive and aquatic therapy, respectively.[27]

Pharmacotherapy

Nonsteroidal anti-inflammatory drugs

NSAIDs are recommended as the first line of treatment in axSpA. They have been shown to be effective in reducing back pain and stiffness. NSAIDs are equally effective in nr-axSpA and AS and there is no clear difference in the effectiveness of different NSAIDs.[28,29] Patients respond in 2 weeks of NSAID therapy and the response rates continue to increase during the first 24 weeks.[30] Long-term NSAID therapy has been a concern and patients should be informed about the potential risks including cardiovascular, gastrointestinal, and renal risk.[28]

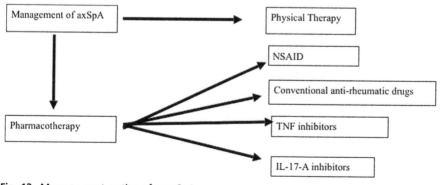

Fig. 12. Management options for axSpA.

Conventional antirheumatic drugs

Conventional antirheumatic drugs, such as methotrexate, sulfasalazine, and leflunomide, have a limited role in peripheral manifestations of axSpA, and are not effective in axial disease.[27]

Tumor necrosis factor inhibitors

TNFi is the main biologic class for the treatment of axSpA after failure of NSAIDs to control the symptoms. There are currently five TNFi available in the United States: (1) infliximab, (2) adalimumab, (3) etanercept, (4) golimumab, and (5) certolizumab. Infliximab and golimumab are the only TNFi that can be given via an infusion, whereas the others are given as subcutaneous injections. All TNFi have been shown to be effective in improving musculoskeletal manifestations of axSpA, reducing CRP levels and levels of inflammation seen on MRI of the sacroiliac joints. Monoclonal antibodies against TNF (adalimumab, certolizumab, golimumab, and infliximab) are more effective for acute anterior uveitis compared with soluble receptor (etanercept). All patients receiving biologic therapy should be screened for hepatitis B, hepatitis C, and tuberculosis.

Interleukin-17A inhibitors

The IL-17 pathway plays a major role in the pathogenesis of axSpA.[31] IL-17A inhibitors are the latest class of biologic medications that have been approved for the treatment of AS. These medications are currently being used in patients who fail to respond adequately to TNFi, or in those who had adverse effects related to TNFi. The IL-17A inhibitor secukinumab was the first medication in this class to be approved for AS, and the response rates of patients on IL-17A inhibitors are close to patients on TNFi therapy. Ixekizumab is the other IL-17A inhibitor that was recently approved for the treatment of axSpA. Bimekizumab (IL-17A and IL-17F inhibitor) is under investigation for AS. Brodalumab (IL-17A receptor inhibitor) is not indicated in AS.

Emerging Therapies

Janus kinase inhibitors are oral therapies that have generated tremendous interest in the last few years as a potential treatment option for axSpA. Although no oral medication is approved for the treatment of AS, there is an ongoing phase 3 trial to evaluate the efficacy of tofacitinib in patients with AS. Tofacitinib is already recommended as a third-line treatment option in patients with active AS in the ACR/SAA/SPARTAN treatment guidelines.[27] Two phase 2 trials looking at the efficacy of upadacitinib and filgotinib in patients with AS were successful.[32,33]

SUMMARY

axSpA includes AS and nr-axSpA. The prevalence of axSpA is estimated to be 1% to 2% in the general population. The diagnosis of axSpA is challenging because one of the cardinal features is back pain, which is common in the general population. That being said, the back pain associated with axSpA is usually inflammatory in nature. It is characterized by buttock pain, morning stiffness, and improvement with exercise and with NSAIDs. Clinicians should be vigilant to pick up peripheral manifestations of axSpA, such as enthesitis and dactylitis. Extra-articular manifestations, such as uveitis, psoriasis, and inflammatory bowel disease, can be the initial presenting feature. There is no blood test to diagnose axSpA. The diagnosis of axSpA is primarily clinical, and imaging modalities, such as radiograph and MRI of the sacroiliac joint, provide valuable supportive information. If there is suspicion for axSpA, patients should be referred to rheumatology because early treatment has shown to improve outcomes in axSpA. New treatment modalities, such as TNFi and IL-17A inhibitor, have had significant impact on axSpA.

CLINICS CARE POINTS

- Back pain lasting for > 3 m with onset prior to 45 years should warrant an evaluation for axSpA.
- Clinicans should be vigilant about extra-articular manifestations of axSpA like psoriasis, enthesitis, uveitis and IBD.
- All patients with axSpA should receive physical therapy and a trial of NSAID's
- TNFi and IL17A inhibitors are approved biologics for the treatment of axSpA.

DISCLOSURE

A. Kumthekar has no disclosures. A. Deodhar has the following disclosures: Consulting, Advisory Boards for AbbVie, Amgen, Boehringer Ingelheim, Celgene, Eli Lilly, Galapagos, Glaxo Smith & Kline, Janssen, Novartis, Pfizer, and UCB. Research Grants from AbbVie, Eli Lilly, GlaxoSmithKline, Novartis, Pfizer, and UCB.

REFERENCES

1. Garg N, van den Bosch F, Deodhar A. The concept of spondyloarthritis: where are we now? Best Pract Res Clin Rheumatol 2014;28(5):663–72.
2. Ahearn JM, Hochberg MC. Epidemiology and genetics of ankylosing spondylitis. J Rheumatol Suppl 1988;16:22–8.
3. van der Linden SM, Valkenburg HA, de Jongh BM, et al. The risk of developing ankylosing spondylitis in HLA-B27 positive individuals. A comparison of relatives of spondylitis patients with the general population. Arthritis Rheum 1984;27(3): 241–9.
4. Reveille JD, Witter JP, Weisman MH. Prevalence of axial spondylarthritis in the United States: estimates from a cross-sectional survey. Arthritis Care Res (Hoboken) 2012;64(6):905–10.
5. Feldtkeller E, Khan MA, van der Heijde D, et al. Age at disease onset and diagnosis delay in HLA-B27 negative vs. positive patients with ankylosing spondylitis. Rheumatol Int 2003;23(2):61–6.
6. Shmagel A, Foley R, Ibrahim H. Epidemiology of chronic low back pain in US adults: data from the 2009-2010 National Health and Nutrition Examination Survey. Arthritis Care Res (Hoboken) 2016;68(11):1688–94.
7. Weisman MH, Witter JP, Reveille JD. The prevalence of inflammatory back pain: population-based estimates from the US National Health and Nutrition Examination Survey, 2009-10. Ann Rheum Dis 2013;72(3):369–73.
8. Danve A, Deodhar A. Axial spondyloarthritis in the USA: diagnostic challenges and missed opportunities. Clin Rheumatol 2019;38(3):625–34.
9. van der Linden S, Valkenburg HA, Cats A. Evaluation of diagnostic criteria for ankylosing spondylitis. A proposal for modification of the New York criteria. Arthritis Rheum 1984;27(4):361–8.
10. Rudwaleit M, Landewe R, van der Heijde D, et al. The development of Assessment of SpondyloArthritis International Society classification criteria for axial spondyloarthritis (part I): classification of paper patients by expert opinion including uncertainty appraisal. Ann Rheum Dis 2009;68(6):770–6.

11. Rudwaleit M, van der Heijde D, Landewe R, et al. The development of Assessment of SpondyloArthritis International Society classification criteria for axial spondyloarthritis (part II): validation and final selection. Ann Rheum Dis 2009; 68(6):777–83.

12. Rudwaleit M, Haibel H, Baraliakos X, et al. The early disease stage in axial spondylarthritis: results from the German Spondyloarthritis Inception Cohort. Arthritis Rheum 2009;60(3):717–27.

13. Vastesaeger N, van der Heijde D, Inman RD, et al. Predicting the outcome of ankylosing spondylitis therapy. Ann Rheum Dis 2011;70(6):973–81.

14. Aggarwal R, Malaviya AN. Diagnosis delay in patients with ankylosing spondylitis: factors and outcomes. An Indian perspective. Clin Rheumatol 2009;28(3): 327–31.

15. Seo MR, Baek HL, Yoon HH, et al. Delayed diagnosis is linked to worse outcomes and unfavourable treatment responses in patients with axial spondyloarthritis. Clin Rheumatol 2015;34(8):1397–405.

16. Rudwaleit M, Listing J, Brandt J, et al. Prediction of a major clinical response (BASDAI 50) to tumour necrosis factor alpha blockers in ankylosing spondylitis. Ann Rheum Dis 2004;63(6):665–70.

17. Sieper J, Rudwaleit M, Baraliakos X, et al. The Assessment of SpondyloArthritis International Society (ASAS) handbook: a guide to assess spondyloarthritis. Ann Rheum Dis 2009;68(Suppl 2):ii1–44.

18. Zeboulon N, Dougados M, Gossec L. Prevalence and characteristics of uveitis in the spondyloarthropathies: a systematic literature review. Ann Rheum Dis 2008; 67(7):955–9.

19. Monnet D, Breban M, Hudry C, et al. Ophthalmic findings and frequency of extraocular manifestations in patients with HLA-B27 uveitis: a study of 175 cases. Ophthalmology 2004;111(4):802–9.

20. Murata KY, Miwa H, Kondo T. Myelin-associated glycoprotein-related neuropathy associated with psoriasis: a case report. J Med Case Rep 2013;7:4.

21. van den Berg R, de Hooge M, Rudwaleit M, et al. ASAS modification of the Berlin algorithm for diagnosing axial spondyloarthritis: results from the SPondyloArthritis Caught Early (SPACE)-cohort and from the Assessment of SpondyloArthritis International Society (ASAS)-cohort. Ann Rheum Dis 2013;72(10):1646–53.

22. Mandl P, Navarro-Compan V, Terslev L, et al. EULAR recommendations for the use of imaging in the diagnosis and management of spondyloarthritis in clinical practice. Ann Rheum Dis 2015;74(7):1327–39.

23. Poddubnyy D, Rudwaleit M, Haibel H, et al. Rates and predictors of radiographic sacroiliitis progression over 2 years in patients with axial spondyloarthritis. Ann Rheum Dis 2011;70(8):1369–74.

24. van Tubergen A, Heuft-Dorenbosch L, Schulpen G, et al. Radiographic assessment of sacroiliitis by radiologists and rheumatologists: does training improve quality? Ann Rheum Dis 2003;62(6):519–25.

25. van den Berg R, Lenczner G, Feydy A, et al. Agreement between clinical practice and trained central reading in reading of sacroiliac joints on plain pelvic radiographs. Results from the DESIR cohort. Arthritis Rheumatol 2014;66(9):2403–11.

26. Ostergaard M, Lambert RG. Imaging in ankylosing spondylitis. Ther Adv Musculoskelet Dis 2012;4(4):301–11.

27. Ward MM, Deodhar A, Gensler LS, et al. 2019 Update of the American College of Rheumatology/Spondylitis Association of America/Spondyloarthritis Research and Treatment Network Recommendations for the Treatment of Ankylosing

Spondylitis and Nonradiographic Axial Spondyloarthritis. Arthritis Rheumatol 2019;71(10):1599–613.

28. Song IH, Poddubnyy DA, Rudwaleit M, et al. Benefits and risks of ankylosing spondylitis treatment with nonsteroidal antiinflammatory drugs. Arthritis Rheum 2008;58(4):929–38.

29. Coxib, traditional NTC, Bhala N, et al. Vascular and upper gastrointestinal effects of non-steroidal anti-inflammatory drugs: meta-analyses of individual participant data from randomised trials. Lancet 2013;382(9894):769–79.

30. Sieper J, Lenaerts J, Wollenhaupt J, et al. Efficacy and safety of infliximab plus naproxen versus naproxen alone in patients with early, active axial spondyloarthritis: results from the double-blind, placebo-controlled INFAST study, Part 1. Ann Rheum Dis 2014;73(1):101–7.

31. Smith JA, Colbert RA. Review: the interleukin-23/interleukin-17 axis in spondyloarthritis pathogenesis: Th17 and beyond. Arthritis Rheumatol 2014;66(2):231–41.

32. van der Heijde D, Baraliakos X, Gensler LS, et al. Efficacy and safety of filgotinib, a selective Janus kinase 1 inhibitor, in patients with active ankylosing spondylitis (TORTUGA): results from a randomised, placebo-controlled, phase 2 trial. Lancet 2018;392(10162):2378–87.

33. van der Heijde D, Song IH, Pangan AL, et al. Efficacy and safety of upadacitinib in patients with active ankylosing spondylitis (SELECT-AXIS 1): a multicentre, randomised, double-blind, placebo-controlled, phase 2/3 trial. Lancet 2019; 394(10214):2108–17.

Psoriatic Arthritis
The Patient and Provider Perspective

Brigitta J. Cintron, DMSc, PA-C

KEYWORDS

- Psoriatic arthritis • Psoriasis • Criteria • Manifestations • Treatment

KEY POINTS

- Psoriatic arthritis (PsA) does not tend to get as much attention as other rheumatic conditions, yet it is not any less burdensome for the patient.
- Use history, imaging, and clinical presentation to help make a definitive diagnosis of PsA.
- Consider the real-life impact for the patient with every disease management decision and when evaluating effectiveness of therapy.

INTRODUCTION

Most providers probably believe that one of the most anxiety-provoking experiences is when you personally become a patient. In the summer of 2012, I found myself in that uncomfortable position. It was not for an acute visit or a brief illness, but rather an experience going from being in the best shape of my life to hardly able to get out of bed without extreme pain. Writing about my patient experiences is not easy for me, but I hope I am a voice for others with similar struggles and bring awareness to the many challenges of psoriatic arthritis (PsA). I began having joint stiffness and pain for no apparent reason. I was so fatigued after working a normal day that I would come home and lay on the couch until bedtime. The initial work-up at my primary care office revealed a significantly elevated erythrocyte sedimentation rate and C-reactive protein. The plan of care was a rheumatology referral. Then began the painful wait for an appointment. Even with two doctors personally calling on my behalf, and being a health care provider myself, it was still 4 months until I could get an appointment with a rheumatologist an hour away. I continued to get worse while I awaited the appointment. I could not continue to work full days. I began even questioning my future. All because out of the blue, I was struck with this rheumatic condition and I needed treatment. I finally saw a rheumatologist in December of 2012. After much bloodwork and ultrasounds, I was diagnosed with PsA. It was mid-January 2013 before my insurance approved therapy with a biologic. In a few

Florida State University, College of Medicine, School of Physician Assistant Practice, 1115 West Call Street, Tallahassee, FL 32306, USA
E-mail address: Brigitta.nuccio@med.fsu.edu

Physician Assist Clin 6 (2021) 149–158
https://doi.org/10.1016/j.cpha.2020.09.007
2405-7991/21/© 2020 Elsevier Inc. All rights reserved.

weeks, I started to get better. After being in such pain and having so much inflammation and stiffness for 6 months, I felt amazing even with mild improvement. Thankfully for me, I continued to get better and better on the biologic. I even called the pharmaceutical company and thanked them for making a drug that gave me my life back. Because of my experience, when it comes to PsA, I understand the patient perspective well.

I was so thankful to finally see a rheumatologist and begin to get better that it did not even bother me at the time that the doctor I saw had terrible bedside manner. One time, I watched the time for our visit and it was literally 6 minutes total from the time I entered the waiting room door, got brought back with the nurse who took vitals, saw the doctor, and came to the check-out counter and exited the office. With all the disease burden in my life, I could have truly benefitted from a bit more attention. A wise man once said when it comes to effective partnerships, "It all starts with a smile" (Ray Keller of Weiner, Arkansas). A smile, handshake, a look in the eye, all of that is truly appreciated by your patient.

As a patient, one thing that causes me a bit of frustration is when providers and others do not understand the disease. So many times, my PsA is referred to as rheumatoid arthritis (RA). PsA is not RA. RA is a terrible disease with its own challenges. Yet, PsA has different pathophysiology and truly deserves its' own recognition. That may seem trivial to some. However, when I was a little girl I had to deal with this awful, itchy, flaky skin and scalp rash. It left me flaking all over the place in constant embarrassment. I had to apply tons of creams and ointments and even coal tar to my scalp with the help of my parents. It got worse and worse. Everyone could see the lesions on my elbows and the flakes in my hair and made fun of me. For these reasons, I insist the PsA is not RA. It is truly a different disease with different pathophysiology and with many other possible manifestations and unique challenges.

In this article I help you relate to your patients with PsA on a deeper level. Knowing the disease process and treatment options is important but understanding the journey for the patient and how it affects their quality of life is paramount for successful remission.

THE STATISTICS

- US prevalence is 0.16% affecting up to 30% of patients with psoriasis[1]
- Age at time of diagnosis is usually between 30 and 50[2]
- The usual order of illness onset is psoriasis followed by PsA 85% of the time, with psoriasis diagnosed at least 10 years prior on average
  - In 5% to 10% of patients PsA presents first and in 5% to 10% PsA and psoriasis present at the same time[1]
- Approximately 15% of patients with psoriasis under the care of a dermatologist have undiagnosed PsA[3]
- PsA has a female/male ratio of 1:1 and is rarely documented among Asians and Blacks[3]
- 47% of patients with PsA develop at least one joint erosion within the first 2 years[1]
- More than half of patients with PsA have five or more deformed joints within 10 years
- A disabling form of PsA develops in approximately 20% of patients over the lifetime of the disease[4]
- First-degree relatives of patients with PsA have a 49 times greater chance of developing PsA compared with the general population[5]

Classification Criteria for Psoriatic Arthritis

In 2006, a study was published that compared the accuracy of current PsA diagnostic criteria and proposed a new classification criteria from the observed data.[6] The result of that publication was the Classification Criteria for Psoriatic Arthritis (CASPAR), which is widely used today. CASPAR criteria are considered to be more highly specific and easier to use than prior criteria.

CASPAR criteria include five major components for the diagnosis of PsA in a patient who is known to have inflammatory musculoskeletal disease (involving the spine, joints, or enthesis). The five components include:

1. Evidence of psoriasis
2. Psoriatic nail dystrophy
3. Negative test for rheumatoid factor
4. Dactylitis
5. Radiographic evidence of juxta-articular new bone formation

Patients receive a score for each component. Any patient with a score of three or higher is considered to have PsA.[3]

The literature also describes key domains of PsA manifestations.[7] These are identified in **Box 1** and then explained in the subsequent sections.

DOMAIN 1: PERIPHERAL ARTHRITIS

- This domain is the most common affecting approximately 95% of patients with PsA.[2]
- Hand and/or feet peripheral joints are plagued with pain, inflammation, and/or tenderness; polyarticular patterns are more often noted compared with oligoarticular.[2]
- All joint digits can be affected, with distal interphalangeal joints being the most common.[1]
- Affected joints may also appear purplish in coloration.[8]

DOMAIN 2: AXIAL DISEASE

- Up to 50% of patients with PsA have axial disease in addition to their peripheral arthritis.[2] Cervical spine disease occurs in 70% of patients with PsA.[9]
- Isolated axial disease only occurs approximately 5% of the time.[2]
- Asymmetric sacroiliitis or spondylitis is the typical presentation.[2]

Box 1
Six key domains of psoriatic arthritis manifestations

1. Peripheral arthritis
2. Axial disease
3. Enthesitis
4. Dactylitis
5. Skin disease
6. Nail dystrophy

- Symptoms may include immobility, restricted range of movement, morning stiffness, atraumatic back pain, and/or sacroiliac joint tenderness. Yet, patients with PsA with spondyloarthropathy often are asymptomatic and disease is found incidentally on radiographs.[2,9]
- On physical examination, restricted cervical rotation, lateral spinal flexion, and chest expansion may be noted; this may also correlate with radiographic evidence of axial disease.[10]

DOMAIN 3: ENTHESITIS

- The area where a ligament, tendon, or joint capsule inserts into a bone and facilitates joint motion is an enthesis. When inflammation occurs at these areas, it is called enthesitis.[11]
- Occurs in 60% to 80% of patients with PsA and leads to a poor prognosis.[12]
- The Achilles tendon and plantar fascia insertion sites and ligament attachments to ribs, spine, and pelvis are most common.[2]
- Soreness, pain, redness, and edema at the insertion site are possible symptoms.[13]
- Younger age, obesity, and more actively inflamed joints are all risk factors for development.[13]
- Quality of life, sleep quality, and functional status are significantly reduced.[12]

DOMAIN 4: DACTYLITIS

- More common in toes and affects approximately 50% of patients with PsA.[3,10,14]
- Often the first notable sign of PsA; may appear months or years before other findings.[14]
- Characteristically called "sausage digits."[8,9]
- Common asymmetric occurrence with edema of an entire digit.[8,9]
- Patients experience a limited range of motion with the edema and pain along the flexor tendons[1] and affected digits are at much higher risk of erosive joint damage.[14]
- In patients with PsA, dactylitis is considered an independent risk factor for cardiovascular morbidity.[14]

DOMAIN 5: SKIN DISEASE

- Known as psoriasis, affected skin areas are thickened, erythematous, and scaly.[10,15]
- Areas most commonly affected in chronic plaque psoriasis include the lumbosacral area; extensor surfaces, such as knees and elbows; the scalp; and intergluteal cleft.[16]
- Scalp and intergluteal or perianal regions have an increased risk of PsA development.[15]
  - Scalp, four times higher risk[17]
  - Intergluteal/perianal, two times higher risk[17]

DOMAIN 6: NAIL DYSTROPHY

- 66% of patients with PsA present with nail lesions.[18]
- Prevalence of disease in the nail matrix may manifest as leukonychia, onychorrhexis, pitting, nail plate crumbling, and red patches on the lunula.

- Nail bed disease is characterized by onycholysis, splinter hemorrhages, subungual hyperkeratosis, and oil spots.[18]

COMORBIDITIES

Unfortunately for the patient with PsA, there are many associated comorbidities.[19] The list, when voiced to the patient, can feel overwhelming and make it seem as if the patient has no chance to remain healthy life long. One patient population studied documented three or more comorbidities among 42% of patients.[20] Please consider your approach when discussing these significant health concerns with your patient with PsA. Comorbidities commonly associated with PsA include:

1. Cardiovascular disease: monitor blood pressure and lipids, calculate risk score, encourage smoking cessation.
2. Obesity: work with your patients to encourage maintaining a healthy weight. Counsel patients on the benefits of weight loss including decreased cardiovascular risk, improved joint health, increased response to therapy, and increased likelihood of remission.[19]
3. Diabetes: check random blood glucose, check hemoglobin A_{1c} at least once for patients older than 45 or when other symptoms or signs indicate necessity.[19]
4. Metabolic syndrome: screen and aggressive work to modify elevated blood pressure, blood glucose, cholesterol, triglycerides, and central obesity. The medical literature regarding the previously mentioned comorbidities includes the following:
   a. One study noted hypercholesterolemia as the comorbidity of the highest incidence, with 61.6% of the study population affected. Obesity was the second highest, with 59.7% affected.[21]
   b. The increased cardiovascular risk, in part, is related to blood processes that contribute to prothrombotic propensity.[22]
   c. Patients with PsA experience an increased burden of inflammation over time, which is associated with increased cardiovascular risk. Patients with psoriasis suffer twice the rate of myocardial infarction than unaffected individuals. Patients who have PsA are at an even higher risk for cardiovascular events than patients who have psoriasis alone.[23]
   d. Patients with PsA have a 30% higher risk of developing diabetes mellitus when treated with topical or oral corticosteroids.[19]
5. Fatty liver disease: consider the risks, benefits, and expectations of medications that cause liver function test abnormalities (eg, methotrexate [MTX], nonsteroidal anti-inflammatory drugs, leflunomide).
6. Inflammatory bowel disease: early referral to gastroenterology for symptoms suggestive of inflammatory bowel disease.
7. Ophthalmic disease: evaluate for symptoms of loss of visual acuity, dry, or red eyes; refer early for further evaluation and comanagement. Potential ophthalmic manifestations include conjunctivitis, scleritis, blepharitis, keratitis, uveitis, and others. Uveitis is the most commonly reported.[19]
8. Depression and anxiety: ask about symptoms, spend the time necessary to address this concern and get patients the help they need:
   a. One study shows patients with PsA exhibiting anxiety and depression at the same incidence rates as diabetes.[21] One would never ignore a comorbid diagnosis of diabetes. With anxiety and depression happening equally as often, more needs to be done to address mental health diagnoses. This study noted a particular rise in the rate of anxiety and depression among females having PsA greater than 2 years.[21]

LABORATORY STUDIES AND IMAGING

There is no definitive laboratory diagnostic test for PsA.[3] It is a clinical diagnosis, requiring the provider to correlate history, physical, and ancillary test results. Laboratory results can assist to rule out other diagnoses.

- 40% of patients with PsA show elevated C-reactive protein and/or erythrocyte sedimentation rate.
- 95% of patients with PsA have a negative rheumatoid factor.
  - If rheumatoid factor is positive, carefully correlate clinical and imaging findings to distinguish PsA from RA.
- 25% of patients with PsA are HLA-B27-positive. However, often this laboratory test is not performed to make the diagnosis because of clinical or historical findings.
- One distinguishing radiographic feature of PsA is bone and cartilage destruction with pathologic new bone formation. Evidence of bone loss with eccentric erosions and joint-space narrowing with new bone formation as noted by bony ankylosis, periostitis, and enthesophytes are often found on peripheral joint radiographs.[24]
- When imaging the axial skeleton, PsA changes to look for include bulky paramarginal and vertical syndesmophytes and unilateral sacroiliitis.
- If an MRI is performed, focal erosions, bone marrow edema, and synovitis may be noted in peripheral and axial structures, especially at entheses. Sacroiliac joint changes may also be noted. MRI is occasionally necessary, when there is a diagnostic dilemma. If your patient suffers from anxiety, please consider the impact of this study on the patient's mental health and well-being. Patients must lie still in a narrow chamber for an extended period of time. It is not a comfortable study to complete.
- Power Doppler ultrasound is gaining in popularity and is a quick, noninvasive way to document enhanced blood flow, tenosynovitis, early erosive disease, enthesophytes, and synovitis.[25]

TREATMENT

Options for PsA are numerous and the list continues to grow as more and more research is completed and new, highly specific drugs become Food and Drug Administration approved. **Fig. 1** lists medication classes currently used to treat PsA and lists nonpharmacologic treatments. Keep in mind that patients may have an extended wait time to be able to see a rheumatology health professional. In primary care, there are some screening laboratory studies and immunizations that you can complete to expedite beginning therapy once they reach the specialist. **Box 2** provides a summary of the screening and vaccination recommendations to consider for those expected to receive pharmacologic treatment of PsA.[26]

These treatments require regular follow-up and monitoring of laboratory parameters. Visit frequency can range from 1 to 6 months depending on success of treatment, need for medication monitoring, stability of laboratory parameters and patient's symptoms, and duration of illness.

The choice of pharmacologic treatment recommendation is based on which anatomic locations are affected by the PsA and the patient's comorbidities. For example, peripheral PsA can respond to nonsteroidal anti-inflammatory drugs and disease-modifying antirheumatic drugs. Axial disease does not tend to respond as well to disease-modifying antirheumatic drugs and biologics tend to work better.

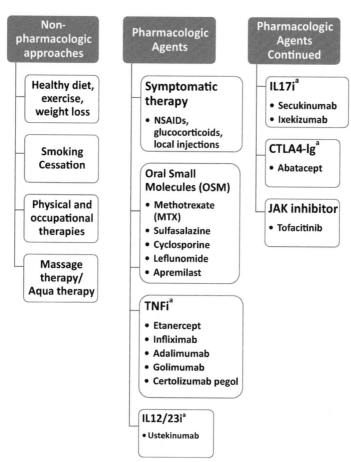

Fig. 1. Overview of available therapies. [a] Biologic medication. CTLA4-Ig, CTLA4-immuno-globulin; IL12/23i, interleukin-12/23 inhibitor; IL17i, interleukin-17 inhibitor; JAK, Janus kinase; NSAIDs, nonsteroidal anti-inflammatory drugs; TNFi, tumor necrosis factor inhibitor. (*Data from* Singh JA, Guyatt G, Ogdie A, et al. 2018 American College of Rheumatology/National Psoriasis Foundation Guideline for the Treatment of Psoriatic Arthritis. Arthritis Rheum. 2019;71(1):5-32. https://doi.org/10.1002/art.40726.)

Patient comorbidities also need to be taken into account. For patients with active PsA and active diabetes, an oral small molecule other than MTX is considered because of increased incidence of fatty liver disease and liver toxicity when using MTX in this patient population. If the patient's diabetes is well controlled or PsA is more severe, then a tumor necrosis factor inhibitor may be considered instead of a non-MTX oral small molecule.[27] For patients with congestive heart failure or demyelinating disease, avoid tumor necrosis factor drugs. For patients with inflammatory bowel disease, avoid interleukin-17 drugs because of risk of exacerbations of the patient's inflammatory bowel disease.

Consider what the target of therapy should be. How much morning stiffness is acceptable to the patient? How many exacerbations are tolerable for the patient, per week, per month? A treat-to-target strategy should be used unless tighter control

---

Box 2
Summary of screening and vaccination recommendations

Hepatitis screening
- Hepatitis B surface antigen
- Hepatitis B core antibody
- Hepatitis B DNA, depending on results of other serologies or in patients with known hepatitis B infection
- Hepatitis C antibody

Tuberculosis screening
- Tuberculosis skin test or interferon-γ release assay

Vaccinations
- Pneumococcal
- Influenza (in season)
- Hepatitis B
- Human papillomavirus (when age appropriate)
- Herpes zoster

---

causes the patient a higher incidence of adverse events, higher cost of therapy, or increased medication burden.[27]

Whether the treatment is pills, injections, infusions, or combinations of these, one must consider how this impacts the patients. Do not forget to incorporate patient education regarding potential side effects and monitoring requirements. Patients should be allowed to express their treatment preference after being well informed of all the potential therapies and the "whole package deal" that goes along with each.

Treatments are often costly and are anticipated to be used long term. Ensure the patient will be able to obtain the medicine before making a prescription choice. If injections must be given, consider if the patient is capable of doing this on his or her own. Does the patient require assistance? Is that assistance available as frequently as the injection must be given? For infusions, will the patient be able to travel to the necessary location or is this a burden the patient cannot endure as frequently as necessary? Often patients must travel great distances to see rheumatology. This leads to more lost work time for people who are often already struggling to meet the demands of a full work schedule because of their condition. How does all this affect the patient's mental health and their family? Is this person also a mother, father, grandmother, daughter, son, or what? Are they able to manage their family and work responsibilities and still maintain their required treatment as they deal with suffering disease burden? Sometimes something as simple as an injection is just too much to handle on a particular day amid all the rest.[19–21]

Patients want to please their providers. They may smile and act as if everything is okay when they are truly crumbling inside. Part of chronic disease management is to ensure the best possible patient well-being. Make sure you take the time to do a proper evaluation and get the patient any extra help they may need. This will decrease many miles and avoid unnecessary detours on the road toward recovery. Patients cannot be in their best physical health if they are not mentally healthy.

SUMMARY

PsA is not RA. It is a unique disease with involvement of the skin, nails, hands, feet, spine, and much more. It commonly occurs in conjunction with anxiety, depression, cardiovascular disease, metabolic syndrome, obesity, diabetes, sleep disturbance, hypertension, hyperlipidemia, and other high-risk conditions. It can seem insurmountable for a patient to manage. Please do not just look at the laboratory studies, imaging, and medications. Please look the patient in the eyes, ask about their true well-being. Help each patient to be able to live the best life possible. Talk with the patient about the management of their disease. Ensure they can manage the challenges of the prescribed therapy. If you are not equipped to handle all of the needs arising from this condition and its comorbidities, partner with other providers who can provide the assistance your patient needs. Remember, "It all starts with a smile."

To come full circle with my patient perspective, I have had PsA for 8 years. I am fortunate and have tolerated my biologic medication without any adverse effects. I receive all the required immunizations and report to the doctor and laboratory studies as advised. I experience infrequent exacerbations of pain. I have a wonderful rheumatologist and Physicians Assistant who listen to all my concerns and want me to be in the best health possible. I work full-time. I have two teenage girls who I run around with all the time to sporting events, school functions, social activities, and so forth. Of course, I get tired like anyone else. My joints hurt if I overdo it. Yet, all in all I cannot complain. I am happy with my treatment and hope, if I can keep my comorbidities low, I will continue to live an active, healthy life for many years to come.

DISCLOSURE

The author has nothing to disclose.

REFERENCES

1. Giannelli A. A review for physician assistants and nurse practitioners on the considerations for diagnosing and treating psoriatic arthritis. Rheumatol Ther 2019; 6(1):5–21.
2. Gottlieb A, Korman NJ, Gordon KB, et al. Guidelines of care for the management of psoriasis and psoriatic arthritis. Section 2. Psoriatic arthritis: overview and guidelines of care for treatment with an emphasis on the biologics. J Am Acad Dermatol 2008;58(5):851–64.
3. Ritchlin CT, Colbert RA, Gladman DD. Psoriatic arthritis. N Engl J Med 2017; 376(10):957–70.
4. Gladman DD, Antoni C, Mease P, et al. Psoriatic arthritis: epidemiology, clinical features, course, and outcome. Ann Rheum Dis 2005;64(suppl 2):ii14–7.
5. De Vlam K, Gottlieb AB, Mease PJ. Current concepts in psoriatic arthritis: pathogenesis and management. Acta Derm Venereol 2014;94:627–34.
6. Taylor W, Gladman D, Helliwell P, et al. Classification criteria for psoriatic arthritis: development of new criteria from a large international study. Arthritis Rheum 2006;54(8):2665–73.
7. Coates LC, Kavanaugh A, Mease PJ, et al. Group for Research and Assessment of Psoriasis and Psoriatic Arthritis 2015 treatment recommendations for psoriatic arthritis. Arthritis Rheum 2016;68(5):1060–71.
8. Busse K, Liao W. Which psoriasis patients develop psoriatic arthritis? Psoriasis Forum 2010;16a(4):17–25.
9. Mok DM. The clinical spectrum and diagnosis of psoriatic arthropathy. Hong Kong Medical Diary 2010;15(5):5–7.
10. Gladman DD. Clinical features and diagnostic considerations in psoriatic arthritis. Rheum Dis Clin North Am 2015;41:569–79.
11. Kaeley GS, Eder L, Aydin SZ, et al. Enthesitis: a hallmark of psoriatic arthritis. Semin Arthritis Rheum 2018;48(1):35–43.

12. Coates LC, Helliwell PS. Psoriatic arthritis: state of the art review. Clin Med (Lond) 2017;17(1):65–70.
13. Polachek A, Li S, Chandran V, et al. Clinical enthesitis in a prospective longitudinal psoriatic arthritis cohort: incidence, prevalence, characteristics, and outcome. Arthritis Care Res 2017;69(11):1685–91.
14. Kaeley GS, Eder L, Aydin SZ, et al. Dactylitis: a hallmark of psoriatic arthritis. Semin Arthritis Rheum 2018;48(2):263–73.
15. Ruiz DG, Azevedo MNL de, Santos OL da R. Psoriatic arthritis: a clinical entity distinct from psoriasis? Rev Bras Reumatol 2012;52(4):630–8.
16. Lebwohl M. Psoriasis. Ann Intern Med 2018;168(7):ITC49–64.
17. Wilson FC, Icen M, Crowson CS, et al. Incidence and clinical predictors of psoriatic arthritis in patients with psoriasis: a population-based study. Arthritis Care Res 2009;61(2):233–9.
18. Sandre MK, Rohekar S. Psoriatic arthritis and nail changes: exploring the relationship. Semin Arthritis Rheum 2014;44(2):162–9.
19. Ogdie A, Schwartzman S, Husni ME. Recognizing and managing comorbidities in psoriatic arthritis. Curr Opin Rheumatol 2015;27(2):118–26.
20. Husted JA, Thavaneswaran A, Chandran V, et al. Incremental effects of comorbidity on quality of life in patients with psoriatic arthritis. J Rheumatol 2013;40(8):1349–56.
21. Khraishi M, Aslanov R, Rampakakis E, et al. Prevalence of cardiovascular risk factors in patients with psoriatic arthritis. Clin Rheumatol 2014;33(10):1495–500.
22. Beinsberger J, Heemskerk J, Cosemans J. Chronic arthritis and cardiovascular disease: altered blood parameters give rise to a prothombotic propensity. Semin Arthritis Rheum 2014;44(3):345–52.
23. Eder L, Thavaneswaran A, Chandran V, et al. Increased burden of inflammation over time is associated with the extent of atherosclerotic plaques in patients with psoriatic arthritis. Ann Rheum Dis 2015;74(10):1830–5.
24. Poggenborg RP, Østergaard M, Terslev L. Imaging in psoriatic arthritis. Rheum Dis Clin North Am 2015;41(4):593–613.
25. Poggenborg RP, Terslev L, Pedersen SJ, et al. Recent advances in imaging in psoriatic arthritis. Ther Adv Musculoskelet 2011;3(1):43–53.
26. Smith B, Nuccio B, Graves K, et al. Preparing patients for biologic medications for dermatologic and rheumatic diseases. J Am Acad Physician Assist 2018;31(6):23–8.
27. Singh JA, Guyatt G, Ogdie A, et al. 2018 American College of Rheumatology/National Psoriasis Foundation guideline for the treatment of psoriatic arthritis. Arthritis Rheum 2019;71(1):5–32.

Systemic Sclerosis: A Comprehensive Approach to Diagnosis and Management

Kristin M. D'Silva, MD*, Marcy B. Bolster, MD

KEYWORDS

- Systemic sclerosis • Scleroderma • Autoimmunity • Vasculopathy • Fibrosis

KEY POINTS

- Systemic sclerosis (scleroderma) is a progressive multisystem disease characterized by autoimmunity, endothelial cell dysfunction, and excessive fibrosis in the skin and internal organs.
- Interstitial lung disease (ILD), pulmonary arterial hypertension, and scleroderma renal crisis are life-threatening manifestations for which screening and early detection are important.
- Pharmacologic treatment is directed at the underlying manifestations of the disease (eg, mycophenolate mofetil for diffuse skin thickening and symptomatic progressive ILD, proton pump inhibitors for gastroesophageal reflux disease, and calcium channel blockers for Raynaud phenomenon).
- Occupational and physical therapy help improve range of motion and function.
- Depression is a common and often overlooked comorbidity, and some patients benefit from antidepressants and/or psychotherapy.

INTRODUCTION

Systemic sclerosis (SSc), also called scleroderma, is a progressive multisystem disease characterized by autoimmunity, endothelial cell dysfunction, and excessive fibrosis. In addition to affecting the skin, SSc can involve the blood vessels, lungs (parenchyma, vasculature), heart, kidneys, gastrointestinal tract, and musculoskeletal system. The clinical features and disease course are variable; treatment strategies are directed toward each patient's specific manifestations.

Skin thickening in SSc typically begins on the fingers and moves proximally. SSc is divided into 2 subsets of cutaneous disease: limited and diffuse. Limited cutaneous

Division of Rheumatology, Allergy, and Immunology, Massachusetts General Hospital, 55 Fruit Street, Bulfinch 165, Boston, MA 02114, USA
* Corresponding author.
E-mail address: kmdsilva@partners.org
Twitter: @kmdsilvaMD (K.M.D.)

Physician Assist Clin 6 (2021) 159–175
https://doi.org/10.1016/j.cpha.2020.09.001
2405-7991/21/© 2020 Elsevier Inc. All rights reserved.

SSc is defined as skin thickening distal to the elbows and knees, whereas skin changes in diffuse cutaneous SSc involve thickening proximal to the elbows and knees. Facial skin involvement can occur in both limited and diffuse SSc. Limited cutaneous SSc was formerly termed CREST syndrome (associated features include calcinosis, Raynaud phenomenon [RP], esophageal dysmotility, sclerodactyly, and telangiectasias); this terminology is no longer commonly used, and these features occur in patients with either limited or diffuse disease.

SSc is a serious progressive disease associated with significant morbidity and mortality. However, survival in SSc has improved in recent years, likely because of earlier diagnosis, earlier identification of disease manifestations, and improvement in therapies. For example, 10-year survival from scleroderma renal crisis (SRC) has increased from less than 10% in the 1970s to 52% to 65% currently with prompt initiation of angiotensin-converting enzyme (ACE) inhibitors in affected patients.[1] Despite these advances, mortality remains high, with up to 22 years of life lost in women and 26 years of life lost in men.[2-4]

Patients with SSc benefit from interprofessional care and multidisciplinary collaboration from rheumatologists, physician assistants (PAs), other medical specialists (such as pulmonologists, gastroenterologists, nephrologists), physical therapists, and occupational therapists to minimize long-term disability and mortality. PAs can play a significant role in educating patients about SSc and its management. This article discusses the pathophysiology, epidemiology, classification criteria, clinical manifestations, evaluation, and treatment of SSc.

PATHOPHYSIOLOGY

Although the pathophysiology of SSc is complex and incompletely understood, it involves autoimmunity, vasculopathy, and fibrosis. Initially, microvascular injury causes endothelial cell activation and platelet aggregation,[5] which results in tissue hypoxia and activation of an inflammatory response, leading to recruitment of lymphocytes and macrophages, which secrete cytokines including, but not limited to, transforming growth factor-β, interleukin-13, interleukin-6, interferon-α, and platelet factor 4.[5,6] As a result of this inflammatory milieu, fibroblasts differentiate into myofibroblasts, which secrete excessive extracellular matrix components resulting in fibrosis.[5]

More than 90% of patients with SSc have a positive antinuclear antibody (ANA) test; in some studies, the prevalence is as high as 98%.[7] There are several SSc-specific autoantibodies associated with various clinical manifestations with considerable overlap between autoantibody profiles and disease manifestations (**Table 1**). Anticentromere, anti-Th/To, and anti–U1-ribonucleoprotein (RNP) antibodies are seen in patients with limited cutaneous SSc and are associated with pulmonary arterial hypertension (PAH). Anti–topoisomerase I (Scl-70) antibody is associated with diffuse cutaneous SSc and ILD. The anti–RNA polymerase III antibody is associated with diffuse cutaneous SSc, SRC, digital ulcers, gastric antral vascular ectasia (GAVE), and malignancy. Antifibrillarin antibody (anti-U3 RNP) is associated with diffuse cutaneous involvement, SRC, and cardiac involvement.[8,9] Other antibodies, such as anti–polymyositis-scleroderma (PM-Scl) antibodies, are associated with overlap syndromes, with manifestations of SSc and other autoimmune diseases such as systemic lupus erythematosus (SLE) and myositis.[5] Mixed connective tissue disease is a diagnosis with established classification criteria that include positive anti-U1-RNP antibodies and clinical features related to 2 or more autoimmune diseases including SSc, SLE, RA, and inflammatory myopathy.[10] In contrast, patients may meet classification criteria for 2 or more

Table 1
Antibodies in systemic sclerosis and common disease-specific associations

Antibody	Cutaneous Involvement	Associations
Anti–topoisomerase I (Scl-70)	Diffuse	• Interstitial lung disease • Cardiac involvement
Anti–RNA polymerase III	Diffuse	• Scleroderma renal crisis • Gastric antral vascular ectasia • Digital ulcers • Malignancy
Antifibrillarin (U3-ribonucleoprotein, U3-RNP)	Diffuse	• Cardiac involvement • SRC
Antipolymyositis/scleroderma (PM-Scl)	Diffuse	• Overlap syndrome with features of SSc and inflammatory myositis
Anticentromere	Limited	• Pulmonary arterial hypertension • Sclerodactyly, telangiectasias, and calcinosis may be prominent features
Anti-Th/To	Limited	• Interstitial lung disease • Pulmonary arterial hypertension • SRC
Anti–U1-ribonucleoprotein	Limited	• Pulmonary arterial hypertension • Mixed connective tissue disease

conditions (overlap syndromes) or may not fully meet classification criteria for any condition (undifferentiated connective tissue disease).

EPIDEMIOLOGY

SSc has a prevalence of 50 to 300 per million people and more commonly develops in women, with a peak age of onset in the fifth decade of life.[2,11] SSc is more common, has onset at a younger age, and tends to have a more severe course in African Americans.[2] For most patients, the cause of SSc is unknown, and there are likely complex interactions between genetic risk factors and environmental exposures. For example, the Choctaw Native Americans in southeastern Oklahoma have a 10-fold increased prevalence of SSc, predominantly having diffuse cutaneous SSc and a positive anti–Scl-70 antibody.[2] A genome-wide association study in this population showed multiple genetic markers associated with SSc, including fibrillin 1 and topoisomerase 1.[2]

CLASSIFICATION CRITERIA

In 2013, the American College of Rheumatology (ACR) and European League Against Rheumatism (EULAR) published SSc classification criteria, which have a sensitivity of 91% and specificity of 92% (**Table 2**).[12] Although designed for enrolling patients in clinical trials, and not intended for use for clinical diagnosis, the criteria provide a helpful guide for distinguishing the primary manifestations of SSc. The classification criteria delineate that skin thickening of both hands extending proximal to the metacarpophalangeal joints is sufficient to classify a patient as having SSc, and patients with skin thickening sparing the fingers are classified as not having SSc.[12] Other fibrosing skin conditions include nephrogenic systemic fibrosis, eosinophilic fasciitis, scleromyxedema, scleredema, graft-versus-host disease, malignancies, and paraneoplastic processes. These

Table 2
2013 American College of Rheumatology and European League Against Rheumatism
Classification Criteria for Systemic Sclerosis

Feature	Number of Points
Skin thickening of the fingers of both hands extending proximal to the metacarpophalangeal joints	9
Finger involvement (only count the highest score):	
Puffy fingers	2
Sclerodactyly[a]	4
Fingertip lesions (only count the highest score):	
Digital tip ulcers	2
Pitting scars	3
Telangiectasias	2
Abnormal nailfold capillaries	2
PAH and/or interstitial lung disease	2
Raynaud phenomenon	3
Scleroderma-related antibodies	3

A score of greater than or equal to 9 classifies a patient as having SSc for clinical trials.
 [a] Sclerodactyly defined as skin thickening between the metacarpophalangeal joints and proximal interphalangeal joints.
Data from van den Hoogen F, Khanna D, Fransen J, et al. 2013 classification criteria for systemic sclerosis: an American College of Rheumatology/European League against Rheumatism collaborative initiative. Arthritis Rheum. 2013;65(11):2737-2747. https://doi.org/10.1002/art.38098.

alternative diagnoses should be considered in patients with skin fibrosis who have a negative ANA, absence of RP, and skin thickening that spares the fingers.[7]

CLINICAL FEATURES
Raynaud Phenomenon

RP, reversible cold-induced color changes caused by vasospasm in the fingers and toes, is typically the first symptom in patients with SSc and is present in approximately 95% of patients (**Fig. 1**).[13] Classically, RP is described as a triphasic color change of the digits: white pallor caused by vasospasm, dusky hue from ischemia, followed by redness from reactive hyperemia. However, many patients do not experience all 3 phases of color changes.

When evaluating a patient with cold-induced color changes of the digits, it is important to establish a diagnosis of RP based on the clinical history, determine whether it is primary or secondary, and evaluate for complications such as digital ulcers. Primary RP is not associated with systemic rheumatic disease and can be seen in 3% to 5% of the general population.[14] Primary RP most commonly occurs in young healthy women, with onset in teens and 20s, and is associated with a negative ANA and normal nailfold capillary examination. Secondary RP occurs in autoimmune diseases such as SSc, dermatomyositis, SLE, rheumatoid arthritis, and Sjögren syndrome. RP in patients with SSc or dermatomyositis is associated with characteristic patterns on nailfold capillaroscopy of capillary dilatation or dilatation with areas of avascularity. Severe RP can lead to complications including digital ulcers (**Fig. 2**A), which can result in dry gangrene (see **Fig. 2**B), autoamputation (see **Fig. 2**A), and secondary infections (see **Fig. 2**C). With prolonged digital ischemia, resorption of the distal phalanges can occur, a process called acro-osteolysis, as shown radiographically (see **Fig. 2**D).[13]

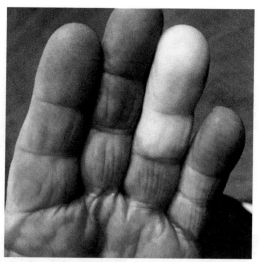

Fig. 1. RP, a reversible cold-induced color change caused by vasospasm in the fingers and/or toes.

Cutaneous Manifestations

Nonpitting digital edema (puffy hands) is often the first non-Raynaud symptom to develop in SSc (**Fig. 3**).[13,15] Sclerodactyly, or skin thickening of the fingers, often follows puffy fingers (**Fig. 4**). Later in the disease, typically approximately 2 years after the onset of skin thickening, the skin may become atrophic and soften. Facial skin thickening can occur in both limited and diffuse disease and can cause a masklike facies with reduced oral aperture, thin lips, and radial furrowing around the mouth resulting in difficulty eating and expressing emotions (**Fig. 5**).[15] Approximately 5% of patients with SSc have no skin thickening (ie, SSc sine scleroderma) but meet classification criteria for SSc.

Other cutaneous manifestations of SSc include calcinosis, telangiectasias, digital pits, and digital ulcers. Calcinosis occurs when calcium-containing salts deposit in the skin and subcutaneous tissues, often involving hands, elbows, pressure points, or other areas exposed to minor trauma (**Fig. 6**).[13] Calcinosis can cause pain, ulceration, and soft tissue infections. Telangiectasias are dilated capillaries that most commonly occur on the mucosal membranes, face, hands, and chest (see **Figs. 2**A and **5**). Calcinosis and telangiectasias occur more commonly in patients with limited cutaneous SSc but can also be seen in those with diffuse disease.

Interstitial Lung Disease

Clinically significant interstitial lung disease (ILD) is more common in diffuse cutaneous SSc (approximately 53% of patients) but can also occur in patients with limited cutaneous SSc (approximately 35% of patients).[2] Patients with ILD may present with progressive dyspnea, dry cough, fatigue, and unexplained weight loss. On physical examination, patients may have tachypnea and basilar Velcro-like crackles.

Many experts obtain baseline pulmonary function tests (PFTs), including spirometry, lung volumes, and diffusion capacity of carbon monoxide (DLCO), high-resolution computed tomography of the chest (HRCT), and an echocardiogram with measurement

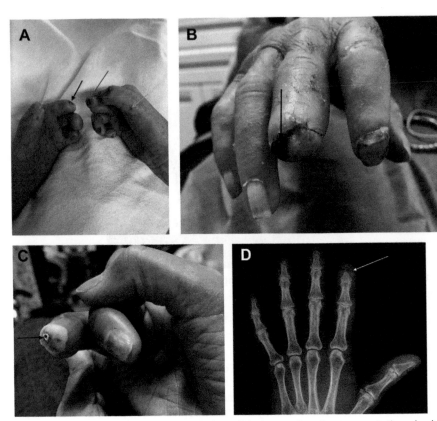

Fig. 2. (*A*) Severe RP resulting in digital ulcers (*black arrow*) and autoamputations (*red arrow*). This patient also has multiple telangiectasias (*green arrow*). (*B*) Digital ulcer with associated dry gangrene (*black arrow*). Of note, there is also autoamputation of the same digit. (*C*) Digital ulcer with superimposed infection (*black arrow*). (*D*) Acro-osteolysis (*white arrow*), resorption of the distal phalanges, seen radiographically, which can occur in patients with SSc.

of the right ventricular systolic pressure (RVSP) to screen for ILD and PAH at the time of diagnosis in all patients with SSc.[16] SSc ILD is characterized by a restrictive pattern on PFTs, with a reduced forced vital capacity (FVC) (<80% predicted) and normal ratio of forced expiratory volume at 1 second to FVC ($\geq$ 70%).[2] An FVC less than 70% predicted and abnormality of greater than 20% of the lung parenchyma on HRCT generally correlate with more severe and symptomatic pulmonary disease.[2]

The most common pattern of lung injury seen on HRCT is nonspecific interstitial pneumonia (NSIP), consisting of ground-glass opacities and reticular changes without frank honeycombing (**Fig. 7**).[2] In addition to lung parenchymal changes, HRCT may show a patulous esophagus because concomitant esophageal disease is common. Some patients may have interstitial lung abnormalities without cough or dyspnea; these patients should be monitored carefully for the development of symptoms. Experts recommend annual PFTs (more frequently as guided by symptoms, presence of recent onset of diffuse skin disease, or anti–Scl-70 antibody positivity), for the first several years after the onset of the first non-Raynaud symptom, because this is the time in which ILD most commonly develops.[2]

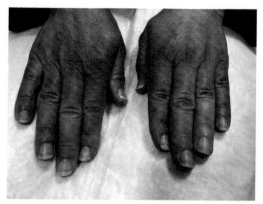

Fig. 3. Nonpitting digital edema (puffy hands) in a patient with early SSc.

Pulmonary Arterial Hypertension

PAH is more common in limited cutaneous SSc but can also be seen in patients with diffuse skin disease. Patients with PAH present with fatigue and dyspnea on exertion. They may also experience lower extremity swelling, dizziness, syncope, chest pain, or palpitations. Physical examination findings include reduced oxygen saturation, increased pulmonic component of the second heart sound, tricuspid regurgitation murmur, and signs of right heart failure, such as increased jugular venous pressure, ascites, and lower extremity edema.

Although PFTs and echocardiogram can suggest the presence of PAH, right heart catheterization (RHC) is the gold standard for diagnosis. On PFTs, a disproportionately low DLCO relative to lung volumes suggests the presence of PAH. On echocardiogram, an estimated RVSP greater than or equal to 35 mm Hg also supports a diagnosis of PAH, although this test is neither sensitive nor specific. In patients in whom PAH is suspected, based on symptoms or diagnostic testing, RHC is the most reliable diagnostic test; a mean pulmonary arterial pressure greater than or equal to 25 mm Hg with a normal pulmonary capillary wedge pressure confirms the presence of PAH.

Gastrointestinal Manifestations

Up to 90% of patients with SSc experience dysmotility of the gastrointestinal tract, possibly caused by microvascular insufficiency causing smooth muscle atrophy,

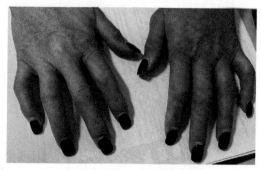

Fig. 4. Sclerodactyly with thickening of the skin of the fingers, resulting in loss of the normal skin folds. Of note, this patient also has flexion contractures of the bilateral fifth digits.

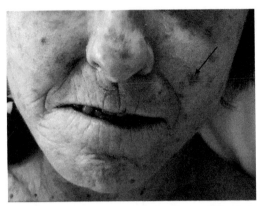

Fig. 5. Facial skin thickening can cause an expressionless masklike facies with reduced oral aperture, thin lips, and radial furrowing around the mouth. Of note, this patient also has several facial telangiectasias (*black arrow*).

although the pathogenesis remains unclear.[17] Any part of the gastrointestinal tract, from the mouth to the anus, can be affected; esophageal involvement is most common, and symptoms commonly include gastroesophageal reflux, dysphagia, and water brash (excess sour-tasting saliva caused by acid reflux).[17] Diagnostic testing may include a barium esophagram showing decreased contractility, esophageal pH monitoring revealing gastroesophageal reflux of acid, and esophageal manometry showing decreased lower esophageal sphincter tone.

Up to 50% of patients may have gastroparesis characterized by symptoms of bloating, nausea, vomiting, early satiety, and unintentional weight loss.[17] Small and large intestinal dysmotility can cause abdominal distention, diarrhea, small intestinal bowel overgrowth, constipation, fecal incontinence, and pseudo-obstruction (dilated bowel

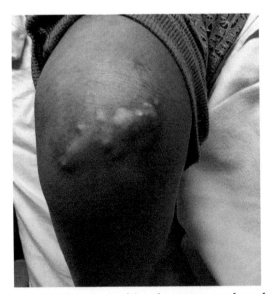

Fig. 6. Subcutaneous calcium deposits overlying the extensor surface of the knee.

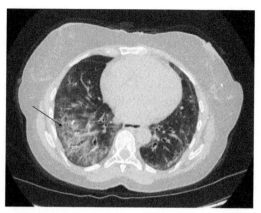

Fig. 7. High-resolution computed tomography of the chest in a patient with SSc, showing NSIP, characterized by a mixture of ground-glass opacities (*black arrow*) and reticular changes, without frank honeycombing.

loops without an anatomic cause, thus not requiring surgical correction). Depression is common in patients with SSc and correlates with more severe gastrointestinal symptoms.[18]

In addition, GAVE is a serious problem of dilated blood vessels in the gastric mucosa that can lead to gastrointestinal bleeding. This condition is associated with positive RNA polymerase III antibodies but can also occur in others. GAVE may cause chronic bleeding leading to iron deficiency anemia or acute bleeding precipitating hemodynamic instability.[19] On upper endoscopy, long parallel dilated blood vessels are visualized in the stomach, giving the characteristic watermelon appearance.[19]

Cardiac Involvement

Cardiac involvement often goes undetected in patients with SSc; it can include cardiac inflammation and/or fibrosis and is a poor prognostic indicator.[20] Patients present with dyspnea, chest pain, syncope, palpitations, and/or lower extremity edema, and it can be difficult to differentiate from pulmonary manifestations. Its pathogenesis may relate to microvascular ischemia and/or myocarditis, and patients can present with heart failure, arrhythmias, pericarditis, and/or pericardial effusions.[20] Risk factors for cardiac involvement include diffuse cutaneous disease, male sex, African American ethnicity, older age at disease onset, tendon friction rubs (discussed later), and myositis.[20]

In evaluating patients for cardiac involvement, an electrocardiogram and echocardiogram should be performed to assess for arrhythmias and structural abnormalities, respectively. In addition, cardiac magnetic resonance imaging can be useful to detect cardiac involvement in SSc, because late gadolinium enhancement can be seen with focal myocardial fibrosis and correlates with heart failure and risk of arrhythmias.[20] Blood levels of brain natriuretic peptide can be both diagnostic and prognostic in PAH and myocardial disease in SSc.[20]

Scleroderma Renal Crisis

SRC, heralded by the onset of hypertension, presents identically to malignant hypertension and may be associated with progressive renal failure, microangiopathic hemolytic anemia, and thrombocytopenia. SRC occurs in approximately 10% of patients with SSc, almost exclusively in patients with diffuse cutaneous SSc.[1] Patients may present with dyspnea, headache, seizures, pulmonary edema, and/or lower extremity edema. Laboratory findings include hemolytic anemia, schistocytes on peripheral blood smear, thrombocytopenia, increased serum creatinine level, and mild proteinuria.

Risk factors for SRC include diffuse skin disease, particularly in patients with rapid progression of skin thickening, large joint contractures, disease duration less than 4 years, tendon friction rubs, positive anti–RNA polymerase III antibody, new-onset anemia, pericardial effusions, and congestive heart failure. Patients at high risk for SRC should be advised to regularly monitor their blood pressure (BP) at home (at least weekly) and notify their provider immediately if hypertensive (or if BP is higher than usual). SRC should be suspected in patients with a systolic BP greater than or equal to 140 mm Hg, a diastolic BP greater than or equal to 90 mm Hg, an increase in systolic BP greater than or equal to 30 mm Hg, an increase in diastolic BP greater than or equal to 20 mm Hg, an increase in serum creatinine level greater than or equal to 50%, proteinuria, or hematuria.[1]

Approximately 10% of patients with SRC may have normal BP, termed normotensive renal crisis, and glucocorticoid use at a dose of prednisone 15 mg daily or higher may be a risk factor.[1] Because of the risk of normotensive SRC, glucocorticoids, especially at high doses, are avoided if possible in patients with SSc. BP, complete blood cell counts, serum creatinine, and urinalysis should be monitored regularly in patients receiving glucocorticoids.[21]

Musculoskeletal Manifestations

Arthralgias and myalgias are common; inflammatory arthritis occurs in only up to 15%, more commonly in patients with diffuse cutaneous disease.[13] Synovitis can be difficult to detect on examination in those with significant skin thickening. Tendon friction rubs, a leathery rubbing sensation detected by the examiner on movement of a joint through its range of motion, can occur in the tendons of the fingers, wrists, and ankles and is characteristic of the presence of, or risk for developing, diffuse cutaneous disease. Fibrosis and inflammation of the skin and subcutaneous tissue can lead to nerve compression causing carpal tunnel syndrome or other nerve entrapment disorders. Joint flexion contractures caused by skin thickening are present in approximately one-third of patients with SSc and can cause significant pain and functional impairment (see **Fig. 6**).[13]

MANAGEMENT
Raynaud Phenomenon

Conservative measures for RP include wearing mittens, avoiding cold exposure, and maintaining core body warmth by dressing in layers and wearing a warm hat. Nicotine and vasoconstrictive medications, such as pseudoephedrine, should be avoided. Calcium channel blockers (CCBs, such as nifedipine or amlodipine) are the first-line treatment of moderate to severe RP.[14,21,22] Patients with continued symptoms or refractory digital ulcers despite CCBs may benefit from a phosphodiesterase-5 inhibitor, such as sildenafil[23] or tadalafil,[24] which have been shown to reduce the frequency and severity of RP attacks. If 1 or 2 fingers are predominantly affected, particularly with digital ulcers, topical nitroglycerin can be applied to the interdigital webs up to 3 times daily, but this medication should not be combined with phosphodiesterase-5 inhibitors given the serious risk of hypotension. A summary of RP treatments is provided (**Table 3**).

Table 3
Treatments for Raynaud phenomenon

Treatment	Examples	Indication	Evidence Level	Side Effects
CCB (dihydropyridine type)	Amlodipine, nifedipine	First line. Decreases frequency and severity of RP attacks	Strong	Hypotension, flushing, peripheral edema
Phosphodiesterase-5 inhibitor	Sildenafil, tadalafil	Second line. Decreases frequency and severity of RP attacks. Helps digital ulcer healing	Strong	Hypotension, headache, chest pain, myalgias, dyspepsia, vision changes, nasal congestion. Cannot combine with nitrates because of risk of hypotension
Endothelin receptor antagonist	Bosentan	Third line. Reduces number of new digital ulcers	Strong	Liver injury, peripheral edema, headache, teratogenicity
Intravenous prostacyclin analogues	Iloprost, epoprostenol	Third line. Helps severe digit-threatening ischemia and digital ulcer healing	Strong	Hypotension, headache, jaw pain, nausea, cough
Topical nitric oxide donors	Nitroglycerin ointment	Apply to interdigital webs to treat vasospasm	Moderate	Headache, hypotension, drug tolerance
Selective serotonin reuptake inhibitors	Fluoxetine	May decrease frequency and severity of RP attacks	Weak	Apathy, lethargy, impaired concentration, insomnia, headache, decreased libido, nausea, diarrhea

In severe cases of threatened digital ischemia, patients may require hospitalization for pain control, consideration of intravenous prostacyclin, and consultation with a hand surgeon regarding chemical (botulinum toxin type A injections) or surgical sympathectomy.[14] Pain control is essential, because pain is vasoconstrictive, thus worsening digital ischemia. Oral or intravenous antibiotics and/or surgical debridement may be warranted for superimposed infections, although instrumentation should be avoided if possible given the risk of poor wound healing.[14]

Cutaneous Manifestations

Patients with diffuse cutaneous SSc, particularly with rapidly progressive skin thickening, may benefit from immunosuppression. Methotrexate has been shown to improve skin thickening in patients with early disease; it may also help inflammatory arthritis, if present.[21] However, methotrexate has not been shown to improve other manifestations of the disease, including ILD. Furthermore, methotrexate can (rarely) cause a drug-induced pneumonitis; therefore, some clinicians avoid methotrexate in patients with significant ILD. As shown by the Scleroderma Lung Studies I and II (discussed later), cyclophosphamide and mycophenolate mofetil, respectively, can improve skin thickness. There is some evidence to suggest that medications such as rituximab,[25,26] abatacept,[27] and tocilizumab[28] may be helpful for cutaneous and musculoskeletal disease; these may be options for select patients unable to tolerate or refractory to conventional therapies.

Treatments for calcinosis are limited and include diligent wound care and avoidance of trauma. Medications such as diltiazem, minocycline, and colchicine have been used with limited and variable success in small case series.[13] Topical or intralesional sodium thiosulfate and surgical debridement may be considered in some cases.[29]

Interstitial Lung Disease

For most patients with symptomatic or worsening ILD (eg, ≥10% decline in percentage of predicted FVC on serial PFTs), immunosuppression is indicated to prevent progression. Early detection and early intervention are imperative for patients with SSc. There have been 2 randomized controlled trials of medications for SSc ILD. The Scleroderma Lung Study (SLS) I compared 1 year of oral cyclophosphamide (CYC) treatment with placebo (and 2 years of follow-up) and showed significant improvement in symptoms, lung function, and skin thickening in patients treated with CYC.[30] However, CYC was associated with more adverse effects, and, importantly, the treatment benefit with CYC was not sustained at 2-year follow-up. The SLS II compared treatment with mycophenolate mofetil (MMF) for 24 months versus oral CYC for 12 months.[31] Although MMF did not show superiority to CYC for improved lung function or skin thickness, MMF was associated with fewer side effects.[30] Therefore, MMF is the first-line agent for treating SSc ILD, followed by changing MMF to CYC if response is insufficient.[22] Rituximab may have efficacy for skin and lung disease, but evidence is mixed.[25,26]

Antifibrotic therapy has been investigated in SSc ILD.[32] Nintedanib, an intracellular tyrosine kinase inhibitor approved for treatment of idiopathic pulmonary fibrosis, was compared with placebo in patients with SSc ILD (at least 10% fibrosis on HRCT).[32] Both groups were permitted standard-of-care therapies (including MMF). At 1 year, the treatment group showed a small but statistically significant slower rate of FVC decline compared with the placebo group. There were no significant differences in skin thickness or quality-of-life outcomes.[32] Gastrointestinal adverse events were more common with nintedanib compared with placebo.[32] The role of nintedanib in the treatment of SSc ILD remains unclear; it may be effective for some patients.[5]

Pulmonary Arterial Hypertension

Management of PAH caused by SSc is similar to the management of idiopathic PAH, with potent vasodilators including phosphodiesterase-5 inhibitors (eg, sildenafil, tadalafil), endothelin receptor antagonists (eg, ambrisentan, macitentan, bosentan), prostacyclin analogues (eg, epoprostenol, treprostinil), and riociguat (a stimulator of soluble guanylate cyclase).[21] Given the need for baseline and monitoring hemodynamic assessments, these patients should be managed in collaboration with a pulmonologist.

Gastrointestinal Manifestations

For gastroesophageal reflux disease, histamine H2 receptor antagonists (H2 blocker), or proton pump inhibitors (PPIs) administered up to twice daily can be helpful, in addition to reflux precautions such as avoidance of food triggers, alcohol, or meals within 3 hours of bedtime.[19] For persistent symptoms, a twice-daily PPI and nightly H2 blocker could be tried. Vigilance for aspiration precautions is required for patients undergoing invasive procedures requiring supine or Trendelenburg positioning to avoid aspiration. For gastroparesis, dopamine-2 receptor antagonists (such as metoclopramide or domperidone) may be helpful, but they can cause side effects such as dyskinesia and cardiac arrhythmias.[17] Small uncontrolled studies have suggested that intravenous immune globulin has efficacy for gastroparesis in SSc.[17] Rifaximin or other intermittent broad-spectrum antibiotic courses (such as ciprofloxacin or metronidazole) can be effective for patients with alternating diarrhea and constipation caused by small intestinal bowel overgrowth. Because of impaired baseline motility, opiates should be avoided in patients with SSc.

For patients with severe symptoms resulting in significant weight loss, oral nutritional supplements, consultation with dietitians, and consideration of total parenteral nutrition are recommended. Given that dysmotility can affect every segment of the gastrointestinal tract, a percutaneous feeding tube may not bypass problematic segments of the gastrointestinal tract and should generally be avoided. For patients with GAVE, repletion of iron stores and consultation with a gastroenterologist for endoscopic interventions are recommended.[19]

Cardiac Involvement

Myocarditis may be treated with glucocorticoids, cyclophosphamide, or MMF, in coordination with a cardiologist for management of hemodynamics.[20] For patients with heart failure from myocardial fibrosis, escalating immunosuppression may not be effective, and collaboration with a cardiologist is essential for developing a heart failure treatment plan.[20] Advanced therapies such as implantable cardioverter-defibrillators should be considered for patients with low ejection fraction, per cardiology society guidelines.[33] Small coronary vessel vasospasm is thought to be an important mechanism of cardiac involvement in SSc; therefore, CCBs may be helpful. β-blockers must be used cautiously, because they may exacerbate RP because of peripheral vasoconstriction. Pericarditis can be treated with judicious use of nonsteroidal antiinflammatory drugs and/or colchicine. Pericardial effusions are generally asymptomatic and rarely require treatment with glucocorticoids or pericardiocentesis unless there has been rapid accumulation or tamponade.[20]

Scleroderma Renal Crisis

In SRC, renal endothelial injury causes decreased renal blood flow resulting in increased renin levels and subsequent hypertension. SRC management involves hospitalization with early institution and rapid uptitration of ACE inhibitors, generally starting with captopril, given its short duration of action, which allows frequent dose adjustments.[1] Rapid gain of BP control is imperative. Importantly, given the acuity of hypertension onset in SRC, rapid BP reduction does not pose risk of relative end-organ ischemia, as may occur with rapidly reducing BP in malignant hypertension. Although the creatinine level may increase after ACE inhibitor initiation, captopril should be continued because the creatinine increase aligns with the natural course of SRC rather than medication toxicity. If hypertension is refractory to captopril, other agents, such as CCBs, labetalol, minoxidil, or nitroprusside, can be considered. Angiotensin receptor blockers may be less effective than ACE inhibitors in SRC.[34]

Given that renal recovery in SRC can occur up to 18 months after onset, ACE inhibitors should be continued even in patients who are hemodialysis dependent. Approximately one-third of patients requiring hemodialysis for SRC are eventually able to discontinue hemodialysis within 1 year with ACE inhibitor therapy.[5] Although previously the leading cause of mortality in SSc, early recognition and treatment with ACE inhibitors have led to significantly improved patient outcomes. Of note, patients with SSc should not be treated prophylactically with ACE inhibitors, because this has been associated with an increased risk of SRC and worse outcomes, possibly because of masking early SRC.[35]

Musculoskeletal Manifestations

If inflammatory arthritis is present, glucocorticoids (prednisone<15 mg daily because of risk for normotensive SRC) can be used to achieve control in the short term. For long-term management, methotrexate is a common steroid-sparing agent[22]; hydroxychloroquine may also be helpful for inflammatory arthritis.[36] Occupational and physical therapy are important modalities to maintain mobility and prevent contractures. Paraffin wax baths provide symptomatic relief and may help improve mobility.[13]

Hematopoietic Stem Cell Transplant

Hematopoietic stem cell transplant (HSCT) as a treatment option deserves special mention. The SCOT (Scleroderma: Cyclophosphamide or Transplantation) trial compared autologous HSCT with 12 monthly infusions of CYC in patients with diffuse SSc.[37] HSCT was superior to monthly CYC in achieving the primary end point, a composite of survival, skin thickness, disability, and quality of life.[37] However, treatment-related mortality was significantly higher with HSCT compared with CYC.[37] For patients with severe or rapidly progressive SSc, referral to an HSCT center with expertise in treatment of patients with SSc is reasonable.

SUMMARY

SSc is a progressive multisystem disorder associated with features of vasculopathy (eg, RP, digital ulcers, telangiectasias, PAH, renal crisis), fibrosis (eg, skin thickening and ILD), and autoimmunity (eg, presence of scleroderma-associated antibodies). Given the systemic and multiorgan nature of the disease, interprofessional and interdisciplinary care with specialists in rheumatology, pulmonary, cardiology, nephrology, and gastrointestinal diseases may be needed. PAs can play a central role in educating patients about SSc and its management. Depression is a common and often overlooked comorbidity, and patients may benefit from antidepressants as well as group and/or individual psychotherapy. Physical therapy and occupational therapy are important to maintain mobility, strength, and function. Early diagnosis and initiation of treatments have led to improved survival in patients with SSc, although SSc continues to be associated with high morbidity and mortality among systemic rheumatic diseases.

CLINICS CARE POINTS

- Patients with systemic sclerosis often present with Raynaud phenomenon, sclerodactyly, and digital ulcers.

- Life-threatening complications of systemic sclerosis include interstitial lung disease, pulmonary arterial hypertension, cardiomyopathy, scleroderma renal crisis, and gastrointestinal bleeding from gastric antral vascular ectasia.
- Conservative measures to preserve body warmth and calcium channel blockers are the first line treatments for Raynaud phenomenon.
- Immunosuppression (mycophenolate or cyclophosphamide) and antifibrotic therapy (nintedanib) are treatments for interstitial lung disease related to systemic sclerosis.

FUNDING

K.M. D'Silva is supported by the National Institutes of Health Ruth L. Kirschstein Institutional National Research Service Award (T32-AR-007258). M.B. Bolster is supported by the Rheumatology Research Foundation (Grant).

DISCLOSURE

K.M. D'Silva has no disclosures. M.B. Bolster has conducted clinical trials for Cumberland and Corbus, is on the advisory board for Gilead, has educational grants from AbbVie, Pfizer, and Amgen, and has investments in Johnson and Johnson.

REFERENCES

1. Bose N, Chiesa-Vottero A, Chatterjee S. Scleroderma renal crisis. Semin Arthritis Rheum 2015;44(6):687–94.
2. Wells AU, Margaritopoulos GA, Antoniou KM, et al. Interstitial lung disease in systemic sclerosis. Semin Respir Crit Care Med 2014;35(2):213–21.
3. Nikpour M, Baron M. Mortality in systemic sclerosis: lessons learned from population-based and observational cohort studies. Curr Opin Rheumatol 2014;26(2):131–7.
4. Hao Y, Hudson M, Baron M, et al. Early mortality in a multinational systemic sclerosis inception cohort. Arthritis Rheum 2017;69(5):1067–77.
5. Allanore Y, Simms R, Distler O, et al. Systemic sclerosis. Nat Rev Dis Primers 2015;1:1–21.
6. Furue M, Mitoma C, Mitoma H, et al. Pathogenesis of systemic sclerosis-current concept and emerging treatments. Immunol Res 2017;65(4):790–7.
7. Schneeberger D, Tyndall A, Kay J, et al. Systemic sclerosis without antinuclear antibodies or Raynaud's phenomenon: a multicentre study in the prospective EULAR scleroderma trials and research (EUSTAR) database. Rheumatology 2013; 52(3):560–7.
8. Kayser C, Fritzler MJ. Autoantibodies in systemic sclerosis: unanswered questions. Front Immunol 2015;6:1–6.
9. Tall F, Dechomet M, Riviere S, et al. The clinical relevance of antifibrillarin (anti-U3-RNP) autoantibodies in systemic sclerosis. Scand J Immunol 2017;85(1):73–9.
10. Alarcon-Segovia D, Cardiel MH. Comparison between 3 diagnostic criteria for mixed connective tissue disease. J Rheumatol 1989;16(3):328–34.
11. Barnes J, Mayes MD. Epidemiology of systemic sclerosis: incidence, prevalence, survival, risk factors, malignancy, and environmental triggers. Curr Opin Rheumatol 2012;24(2):165–70.
12. Van Den Hoogen F, Khanna D, Fransen J, et al. 2013 Classification criteria for systemic sclerosis: An American College of Rheumatology/European League

Against Rheumatism collaborative initiative. Arthritis Rheum 2013;65(11): 2737–47.

13. Young A, Namas R, Dodge C, et al. Hand impairment in systemic sclerosis: Various manifestations and currently available treatment. Curr Treatm Opt Rheumatol 2016;2(3):252–69.

14. Khouri C, Lepelley M, Bailly S, et al. Comparative efficacy and safety of treatments for secondary Raynaud's phenomenon: a systematic review and network meta-analysis of randomised trials. Lancet Rheumatol 2019;1(4):e237–46.

15. Krieg T, Takehara K. Skin disease: a cardinal feature of systemic sclerosis. Rheumatology 2009;48(Supplement 3):iii14–8.

16. Hoffmann-Vold AM, Fretheim H, Halse AK, et al. Tracking impact of interstitial lung disease in systemic sclerosis in a complete nationwide cohort. Am J Respir Crit Care Med 2019;200(10):1258–66.

17. McMahan ZH, Hummers LK. Gastrointestinal involvement in systemic sclerosis: diagnosis and management. Curr Opin Rheumatol 2018;30(6):533–40.

18. Nietert PJ, Mitchell HC, Bolster MB, et al. Correlates of depression, including overall and gastrointestinal functional status, among patients with systemic sclerosis. J Rheumatol 2005;32(1):51–7.

19. McFarlane IM, Bhamra MS, Kreps A, et al. Gastrointestinal manifestations of systemic sclerosis. Rheumatology (Sunnyvale) 2018;08(01):1–35.

20. Rangarajan V, Matiasz R, Freed BH. Cardiac complications of systemic sclerosis and management: recent progress. Curr Opin Rheumatol 2017;29(6):574–84.

21. Kowal-Bielecka O, Fransen J, Avouac J, et al. Update of EULAR recommendations for the treatment of systemic sclerosis. Ann Rheum Dis 2017;76(8):1327–39.

22. Fernández-Codina A, Walker KM, Pope JE. Treatment algorithms for systemic sclerosis according to experts. Arthritis Rheum 2018;70(11):1820–8.

23. Fries R, Shariat K, von Wilmowsky H, et al. Sildenafil in the treatment of Raynaud's phenomenon resistant to vasodilatory therapy. Circulation 2005;112(19):2980–5.

24. Shenoy PD, Kumar S, Jha LK, et al. Efficacy of tadalafil in secondary Raynaud's phenomenon resistant to vasodilator therapy: a double-blind randomized crossover trial. Rheumatology 2010;49(12):2420–8.

25. Jordan S, Distler JH, Maurer B, et al. Effects and safety of rituximab in systemic sclerosis: an analysis from the European Scleroderma Trial and Research (EUSTAR) group. Ann Rheum Dis 2015;74(6):1188–94.

26. Elhai M, Boubaya M, Distler JH, et al. Outcomes of patients with systemic sclerosis treated with rituximab in contemporary practice: a prospective cohort study. Ann Rheum Dis 2019;78:979–87.

27. Khanna D, Spino C, Johnson S, et al. Abatacept in early diffuse cutaneous systemic sclerosis: results of a phase II investigator-initiated, multicenter, double-blind, randomized, placebo-controlled trial. Arthritis Rheum 2020;72(1):125–36.

28. Khanna D, Denton CP, Jahreis A, et al. Safety and efficacy of subcutaneous tocilizumab in adults with systemic sclerosis (faSScinate): a phase 2, randomised, controlled trial. Lancet 2016;387(10038):2630–40.

29. Ma JE, Ernste FC, Davis MDP, et al. Topical sodium thiosulfate for calcinosis cutis associated with autoimmune connective tissue diseases: the Mayo Clinic experience, 2012–2017. Clin Exp Dermatol 2019;44(5):e189–92.

30. Tashkin DP, Elashoff R, Clements PJ, et al. Cyclophosphamide versus placebo in scleroderma lung disease. N Engl J Med 2006;354(25):2655–66.

31. Tashkin DP, Roth MD, Clements PJ, et al. Mycophenolate mofetil versus oral cyclophosphamide in scleroderma-related interstitial lung disease (SLS II): a

randomised controlled, double-blind, parallel group trial. Lancet Respir Med 2016;4(9):708–19.

32. Distler O, Highland KB, Gahlemann M, et al. Nintedanib for systemic sclerosis-associated interstitial lung disease. New Engl J Med 2019;380(26):2518–28.

33. Yancy CW, Jessup M, Bozkurt B, et al. 2013 ACCF/AHA guideline for the management of heart failure. J Am Coll Cardiol 2013;62(16):e147–239.

34. Caskey F, Thacker E, Johnston P, et al. Failure of losartan to control blood pressure in scleroderma renal crisis. Lancet 1997;349(9052):620.

35. Gordon SM, Hughes JB, Nee R, et al. Systemic sclerosis medications and risk of scleroderma renal crisis. BMC Nephrol 2019;20(1):1–7.

36. Bruni C, Praino E, Guiducci S, et al. Hydroxychloroquine and joint involvement in systemic sclerosis: Preliminary beneficial results from a retrospective case-control series of an EUSTAR center. Joint Bone Spine 2017;84(6):747–8.

37. Sullivan KM, Goldmuntz EA, Keyes-Elstein L, et al. Myeloablative autologous stem-cell transplantation for severe scleroderma. N Engl J Med 2018;378(1):35–47.

Overview of Pediatric Rheumatology: Part One

Heather Benham, DNP, APRN, CPNP-PC[a],*, Tracey B. Wright, MD[b]

KEYWORDS

- Juvenile arthritis • Hypermobility • Scleroderma

KEY POINTS

- The care of children with rheumatic diseases is affected by considerations for growth and development, psychosocial implications, and family dynamics.
- Although there are forms of juvenile idiopathic arthritis that have some equivalency to adult forms of arthritis, it is important to understand the subtypes and complications that are unique in childhood.
- Localized scleroderma is far more common in childhood than systemic sclerosis.

INTRODUCTION

It is estimated that approximately 300,000 children in the United States have juvenile idiopathic arthritis (JIA), the most common pediatric rheumatic disease.[1] This review highlights rheumatic diseases that are unique to children as well as emphasizes how some rheumatic diseases may differ in the pediatric population.

Most pediatric rheumatic diseases are characterized by chronic inflammation, which may negatively affect growth and development without appropriate treatment. Patients may experience local growth disturbances from inflammation within a joint (ie, temporomandibular joint arthritis)[2] as well as more diffuse growth disturbances from systemic inflammation. In addition, chronic glucocorticoid use, a mainstay of treatment of many pediatric rheumatic diseases, is harmful to growth.[3] Glucocorticoids directly suppress growth by inhibiting cell growth and division and production of insulinlike growth factor.[4] Glucocorticoids also increase the differentiation of osteoclasts and decrease differentiation of osteoblasts, resulting in osteopenia.[5] These effects are especially important for youth, as approximately 40% to 60% of adult bone mass is accrued during adolescence with approximately 90% of peak bone mass accrual by 18 years of age.[6] Consequently, harm to bone development during

[a] Pediatric Rheaumtology, Scottish Rite Hospital, 2222 Welborn Street, Dallas, TX 75219, USA;
[b] Division of Rheumatology, Department of Pediatrics, UT Southwestern Medical Center, 5323 Harry Hines Boulevard, MC 9063, Dallas, TX 75390, USA
* Corresponding author.
E-mail address: heather.benham@tsrh.org

Physician Assist Clin 6 (2021) 177–191
https://doi.org/10.1016/j.cpha.2020.09.004
2405-7991/21/© 2020 Elsevier Inc. All rights reserved.

childhood and adolescence has long-lasting, detrimental effects well into adulthood including increased risk of severe osteoporosis and fractures.[6]

Chronic rheumatic disease and its treatment may also negatively affect psychosocial development. Altered appearance due to persistent skin changes from systemic lupus erythematosus or localized scleroderma or significant weight gain and changes in fat distribution from chronic glucocorticoid use can be distressing.[7] In addition, the diagnosis is frequently made during a period of time when children and adolescents are developing their identity and planning for the future.[8]

With earlier diagnosis and improved treatment, children and adolescents diagnosed with rheumatic disease are more likely to survive into adulthood.[9] Thus, attention to the long-term impact of chronic disease and its therapies is even more critical. Children are at risk of developing morbidity and mortality associated with rheumatic disease including malignancy and cardiovascular disease.[10,11] These patients will ultimately transition to adult care and certain "vulnerable" populations are at high risk of experiencing poor outcomes when the transition to adult care does not go well.[8] Beyond knowing their disease course, pediatric patients must learn to navigate the medical system and learn how to self-administer medications.[12]

The care of children must occur in the context of the family. Beyond the provision of financial support and legal consent, the family provides important components of the history, may be involved in medication administration, and helps with medication adherence and coping with chronic illness. In partnership with the family and primary care physician, multidisciplinary care with input from other subspecialists is critical to provide comprehensive care for these children with rheumatic disease.

In the past decade, a rapid development of new knowledge of disease pathophysiology, diagnostics, and therapeutic approaches has occurred. The Childhood Arthritis and Rheumatology Research Alliance (CARRA), the pediatric rheumatology research network in North America, has facilitated the study of pediatric rheumatic disease in a collaborative fashion.[13] CARRA's extensive patient registry of the common pediatric rheumatic diseases improves our ability to understand clinical course and outcomes. The registry has also permitted the development of consensus treatment plans to enable comparative effectiveness research, as it is challenging to perform robust clinical trials for children with rare diseases.[14,15]

JUVENILE IDIOPATHIC ARTHRITIS

JIA is a heterogeneous set of diseases with the hallmark of persistent arthritis in a joint or set of joints lasting for at least 6 weeks, with onset before 16 years of age.[16] Although the exact cause is unknown, these diseases likely occur in a genetically susceptible host and are brought on by an environment trigger. Of course, in childhood JIA is a diagnosis of exclusion. Thus, it is very important to evaluate for other possible causes of arthritis such as infection (local or systemic), malignancy, trauma, or other connective tissue diseases.[17]

Incidence and prevalence rates of JIA vary by gender, race, geographic location, and diagnostic criteria used.[18] A recent study of a managed care population in the United States revealed an incidence rate of 11.9 per 100,000 person-years and a prevalence rate of 44.7 per 100,000 persons.[19]

JIA is an umbrella term that encompasses several subtypes of chronic arthritis. The classification of JIA currently follows the International League of Associations for Rheumatology (ILAR) criteria as a means to standardize nomenclature within the clinical setting and research protocols[20] (**Table 1**). The specific subtype is determined by number of joints involved at onset but also by considerations of axial

Table 1
Juvenile idiopathic arthritis subtypes based on International League of Associations for Rheumatology criteria

Subtypes	Characteristics
Systemic arthritis **(Fig. 2)**	Arthritis in one or more joints, daily fever x 2 wk with one or more of the following: evanescent rash, lymphadenopathy, HSM, or serositis
Oligoarthritis **(Fig. 3)**	Arthritis in 1–4 joints for the first 6 mo of disease. Subtypes: (1) persistent—no more than 4 joints during disease course or (2) extended—affects more than 4 joints after first 6 mo of disease
Polyarthritis (RF−)	Arthritis in 5 or more joints during first 6 mo of disease. RF test negative.
Polyarthritis (RF+)	Arthritis in 5 or more joints during first 6 mo of disease. RF test positive x 2 at least 3 mo apart
Psoriatic arthritis	Arthritis and psoriasis or arthritis and 2 of the following: dactylitis, nail pitting, psoriasis in first-degree relative
Enthesitis-related arthritis	Arthritis with enthesitis or with at least 2 of the following: (1) sacroiliac tenderness and/or inflammatory lumbosacral pain, (2) +HLA-B27, (3) onset in boys older than 6 y, or (4) hx of AS, ERA, sacroiliitis with IBD, Reiter syndrome, or acute anterior uveitis in first-degree relative
Undifferentiated arthritis	Arthritis that fulfils criteria in no category on in 2 or more other categories

Abbreviations: AS, ankylosing spondylitis; ERA, enthesitis-related arthritis; HLA, human leukocyte antigen; HSM, hepatosplenomegaly; hx, history of; IBD, inflammatory bowel disease; RF, rheumatoid factor.

Data from Petty RE, Southwood TR, Manners P, et al. International League of Associations for Rheumatology classification of juvenile idiopathic arthritis: second revision, Edmonton, 2001. The Journal of rheumatology 2004;31:390-2.

involvement, associated rashes and/or fevers, organ involvement, and constitutional symptoms.[21] As the ILAR criteria are imperfect, there have been recent efforts to eliminate the distinctive joint counts as well as identify juvenile-onset subtypes with some equivalency to those seen in adulthood while distinguishing those that are truly unique to children.[22] However, more recent research does highlight the ongoing importance of recognizing patterns and localizations of joint involvement, as this may give insight into disease progression and prognosis, ultimately informing treatment decisions.[23]

Each subtype has a variable presentation, trajectory of disease as well as scope of outcomes and complications.[21] When approaching a child, who may have JIA, in the clinical setting, it is important to obtain a comprehensive history, including assessment for joint pain, swelling, morning stiffness, fever, rashes, changes in activity level, and regression of developmental milestones. Patients with JIA and their parents often deny pain or visible swelling, so a thorough joint examination is crucial. An important distinction in the assessment of JIA compared with adult onset arthritis is the definition for a clinically active joint. In children, this is defined as a joint either with (1) a palpable effusion with or without limitation or pain or (2) a limited joint, without effusion, that is painful to range or tender to palpation.[24] Severe pain or associated erythema to the joint is uncommon in JIA and should raise the concern for septic arthritis or other infectious causes, that is, rheumatic fever.[25]

There is no single laboratory test or set of laboratory tests that are specific for the diagnosis of JIA. Children presenting with a positive antinuclear antibody (ANA) or rheumatoid factor (RF) and musculoskeletal pain but no clinical evidence of an inflammatory arthritis are a low risk for developing JIA.[26–28] It is estimated that the ANA can be positive in nearly 20% of healthy children.[29] Only about 5% of children with JIA have an RF and antibodies targeting citrullinated peptides. These children typically present at an older age, often in adolescence, and have increased risk for erosive disease.[30] It is important to use basic laboratory tests, including complete blood count (CBC), erythrocyte sedimentation rate, and albumin, and often imaging, such as radiograph, ultrasound, and MRI, to help evaluate for other potential causes of joint swelling.[31]

In the context of a JIA diagnosis, it is important to know ANA status in order to determine risk for uveitis and frequency of ophthalmologic evaluations. Approximately 20% of patients with JIA will develop uveitis.[32,33] Those children, who present before the age of 7 years, are early on in their disease course, have an oligoarticular or polyarticular subtype, and have a positive ANA, are at highest risk for chronic uveitis, a form that is often asymptomatic, and should be screened every 3 months for the first 4 years of their disease.[34–37] Similar to the adult-onset equivalents, children with enthesitis-related arthritis, spondyloarthropathies, and psoriatic arthritis are at risk for acute episodes of uveitis.[38,39]

As with adult-onset arthritis, the American College of Rheumatology (ACR) has established a core set of variables used to define disease activity in JIA and monitor response to therapy.[40] The Juvenile Arthritis Disease Activity Score is also used to define level of disease activity (low, moderate, high) and can be quickly calculated in the clinical setting in order to guide treatment decisions.[41,42] The current definition of inactive disease (ID) has led to criteria for clinical remission on medications (ID for minimum of 6 continuous months) and clinical remission off medications (ID for a minimum of 12 continuous months).[43,44] To note, there are current efforts to revise the core set of outcome measures in JIA, incorporating the input of patients and caregivers.[45]

Early, aggressive treatment is essential in JIA, as many children present at a young age, and chronic arthritis can have significant effects on growth and development as well as the health of individual joints. Children with systemic onset JIA, due to increased systemic inflammation and greater need for steroid therapy, have higher risk for overall growth retardation and lower bone density.[46] Those with a persistently active knee or hip are at increased risk for joint contracture and leg length discrepancy.[47,48] Chronic, uncontrolled arthritis can also cause bony overgrowth, joint space narrowing, loss of articular cartilage, and erosions.[49] Arthritis of the TMJ can cause condylar deformities and micrognathia (**Fig. 1**), often leading to long-term functional difficulties.[50,51] Involvement of the cervical spine can lead to malalignment, ankyloses, and narrowing of the spinal canal.[52]

Although an extensive discussion about the treatment of JIA is beyond the scope of this article, there are some important points to discuss. The ACR has published several guidelines on the treatment of JIA and JIA-associated uveitis,[37,53,54] with additional updates expected in 2021. Recent guidelines have considered parent and patient preferences as well as the importance of adjunctive treatments, including physical and occupational therapy. With the introduction of biological medications, there has been an increase in the frequency of inactive disease and low disease activity states as well as decrease in disease damage indices.[55] Achieving these low disease states, particularly in those children with newly diagnosed polyarticular JIA, seems to be affected by early introduction of these agents.[56] In addition, delay in treatment has been associated with a more severe disease course and lower chance for the achievement of remission.[57] Thus, prompt referral to a pediatric rheumatology team is essential.

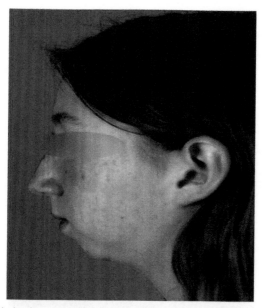

Fig. 1. Micrognathia in the context of Juvenile Idiopathic Arthritis.

MIMICKERS OF JUVENILE IDIOPATHIC ARTHRITIS IN CHILDREN

When considering the diagnosis of JIA in the differential, it is important to remember that there are many other conditions in childhood that can cause joint pain and transient or chronic joint swelling. Benign joint hypermobility (**Fig. 4**) can lead to localized or diffuse joint pain, particularly after periods of increased physical activity.[58,59] In

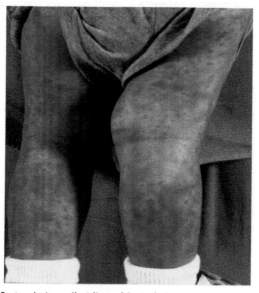

Fig. 2. The rash of Systemic Juvenile Idiopathic Arthritis.

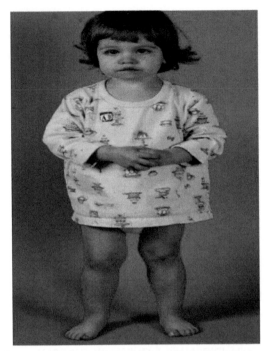

Fig. 3. Oligoarticular Juvenile Idiopathic Arthritis patient with right knee swelling.

addition, children can develop a variety of overuse injuries including apophysitis (ie, Osgood-Schlatter and Sever diseases) and patellofemoral syndrome.[60,61] In the case of acute hip pain with limp, consider transient (toxic) synovitis.[62] When a child reports pain in the lower extremity that is more severe at night and during periods of inactivity, evaluate for osteoid osteoma.[63] Joint swelling, particularly of the knee, could be a form of abnormal synovial proliferation such as pigmented villonodular synovitis or lipoma arborescens.[64,65] Finally, children with leukemia can present with

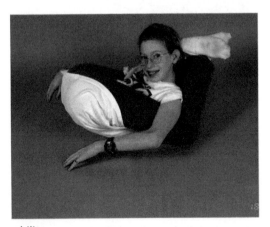

Fig. 4. Joint hypermobility.

arthritis but often have pain out of proportion to physical findings as well as constitutional symptoms such as fever and pallor.[66]

LOCALIZED SCLERODERMA

As systemic sclerosis in adults has been reviewed in detail in an earlier chapter of this journal, the authors focus on localized scleroderma, the form that is 6 to 10 times more common in children.[67] Briefly, juvenile systemic sclerosis (jSSc) is estimated to occur in 0.27 per million children per year,[68] with mean age of onset of 8 to 11.[67] Provisional classification criteria have been developed[69] and in addition to the diagnostic cutaneous changes, clinical manifestations can include Raynaud, arthritis, myositis, gastrointestinal changes, and cardiopulmonary complications. Renal involvement is seen in less than 5% of patients with jSSc.[70] Prognosis is more favorable, with one study showing survival at 10 years of 98% compared with 75% in those with adult onset disease.[71] Death is often attributed to cardiac failure, less often respiratory or renal failure, and increased risk factors have been identified including fibrosis on chest radiograph, increased creatinine levels, and pericarditis.[70] Shorter disease duration at the time of diagnosis has been found to increase survival rates,[70] thus emphasizing the importance of early recognition and prompt referral to a pediatric rheumatologist.

Turning to juvenile localized scleroderma (jLS), although it shares similar pathogenic processes with jSSc, it likely represents a different disease without fibrosis of internal organs.[67,72] Estimated annual incidence rate is 1 to 3 per 100,000 children.[73] Mean age of onset is typically between 7 and 8 years, with a female predominance.[68,74–76] Pathogenesis involves immune disregulation[77] with abnormalities in fibroblasts and vascular elements causing a progressive cascade from inflammation to fibrosis to atrophy.[78]

The current classification of jLS developed by the Pediatric Rheumatology European Society includes 5 subtypes (**Table 2**).[79] Most of the children present with a linear subtype[68,75,80] (**Fig. 5**) with lesions following Blaschko lines, which trace the migration of embryonic cells during development.[67] Active lesions are typically erythematous with violaceous color change, tactile warmth, and abnormal skin texture (smooth, shiny, and/or waxy appearance), whereas chronic changes include dyspigmentation as well as dermal and subcutaneous atrophy.[67] The depth of lesions vary and can affect the dermis, subcutaneous tissue, muscle, and bone. Diagnosis is determined by clinical presentation, as routine bloodwork, including CBC, chemistries, and inflammatory markers, are typically normal.[81] Although the incidence of certain autoantibodies (SCL-70, anticentromere, anti RP11) in jLS is low,[74,82] their presence may indicate risk for deeper tissue involvement, as evidenced by increased incidence of joint contracture and nerve entrapment.[83]

An important subtype of jLS to recognize is en coup de sabre, a form that can affect the face, neck, and scalp (**Fig. 6**). Because of the location of the lesions, in addition to progressive facial atrophy and alopecia, extracutaneous manifestations can include neurologic symptoms, such as headaches and seizures, ocular involvement, and abnormalities of the oral cavity and dentition.[84–86] Therefore, specific recommendations related to the frequency of brain MRI, eye screenings, and dental assessments have been published.[87]

Children with jLS should be followed closely by a pediatric rheumatologist, who can monitor disease activity and assess for damage. In addition to completion of a comprehensive history and focused clinical examination, standardized assessment tools have been developed, the most common being the Localized Scleroderma Cutaneous Assessment Tool,[88] which includes 2 separate measures, an activity score, the

Table 2
Preliminary proposed classification of juvenile localized scleroderma

Main Group	Subtype	Description
Circumscribed	Superficial	Oval or round circumscribed areas of induration limited to the epidermis and dermis, often with altered pigmentation and violaceous, erythematous halo (lilac ring). They can be single or multiple.
	Deep	Oval or round circumscribed deep induration of the skin involving subcutaneous tissue extending to fascia and may involve underlying muscle. The lesions can be single or multiple. Sometimes the primary site of involvement is in the subcutaneous tissue without involvement of the skin.
Linear	Trunk/limbs	Linear induration involving dermis, subcutaneous tissue, and sometimes muscle and underlying bone and affecting the limbs and the trunk.
	Head	En coup de sabre (ECDS). Linear induration that affects the face and the scalp and sometimes involves muscle and underlying bone.
		Parry-Romberg syndrome or progressive hemifacial atrophy loss of tissue on one side of the face that may involve the dermis, subcutaneous tissue, muscle, and bone. The skin is mobile.
Generalized morphea		Induration of the skin starting as individual plaques (4 or more and larger than 3 cm) that become more confluent and involve at least 2 out of 7 anatomic sites (head-neck, right upper extremity, left upper extremity, right lower extremity, left lower extremity, anterior trunk, posterior trunk).
Pansclerotic morphea		Circumferential involvement of limb affecting the skin, subcutaneous tissue, muscle, and bone. The lesion may also involve other areas of the body without internal organs involvement.
Mixed morphea		Combination of 2 or more of the previous subtypes. The order of the concomitant subtypes, specified in brackets, will follow their predominant representation in the individual patient (ie, mixed morphea (linear-circumscribed).

Reprinted with permission from Laxer RM, Zulian F. Localized scleroderma. Current opinion in Rheumatology 2006; 18:606-613.

modified Localized Scleroderma Severity Skin Index (mLoSSI), and a damage score, the modified Localized Scleroderma Damage Index. The mLoSSI, along with Physician Global Assessment-Activity, demonstrates correlation to clinical change (active to inactive) and can help determine response to systemic therapy.[88] In addition, the utility of imaging modalities, such as infrared thermography, ultrasound, and MRI, has been explored and can be beneficial when applying appropriate clinical correlation.[89]

In terms of treatment, recent consensus recommendations have been published, recognizing the efficacy of systemic steroids (oral or intravenous) in combination with methotrexate.[90] Mycophenolate mofetil has also been used, typically in those unresponsive or intolerant to methotrexate[91,92]; however, it may be used in combination with methotrexate as well.[93] Once achieving inactive disease, children with jLS need to

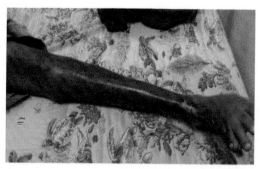

Fig. 5. Linear scleroderma.

be monitored closely, as one recent study demonstrated a relapse rate of 45%, with an average time to relapse of 21 months after discontinuation of therapy.[94]

Referral to a specialist is often delayed, with median time from initial symptoms to definitive diagnosis being 11 months,[80,95] whereas a delay of greater than 2 years can be seen in nearly 20% of children with jLS.[76] Growth differences, including limb girth and length differences as well as facial and truncal hemiatrophy, can be found in nearly 50% of patients.[93] Impaired function is more common in children with muscle atrophy,

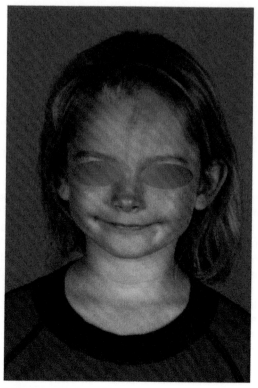

Fig. 6. En Coup de Sabre.

joint contracture, and extremity shortening.[76] Thus, early recognition and referral is essential.

SUMMARY

Part 1 of this review of pediatric rheumatic diseases has addressed general management considerations as well as a review of JIA and jLS. Part 2 continues the discussion of the conditions most commonly seen by pediatric rheumatology providers including systemic lupus, juvenile dermatomyositis, vasculitidies, and autoinflammatory syndromes. A final summary is also included.

DISCLOSURE

The authors have nothing to disclose.

REFERENCES

1. Helmick CG, Felson DT, Lawrence RC, et al. Estimates of the prevalence of arthritis and other rheumatic conditions in the United States. Part I. Arthritis Rheum 2008;58:15–25.
2. Twilt M, Schulten AJ, Nicolaas P, et al. Facioskeletal changes in children with juvenile idiopathic arthritis. Ann Rheum Dis 2006;65:823–5.
3. Rygg M, Pistorio A, Ravelli A, et al. A longitudinal PRINTO study on growth and puberty in juvenile systemic lupus erythematosus. Ann Rheum Dis 2012;71:511–7.
4. Bennett AE, Silverman ED, Miller JJ 3rd, et al. Insulin-like growth factors I and II in children with systemic onset juvenile arthritis. J Rheumatol 1988;15:655–8.
5. Canalis E, Delany AM. Mechanisms of glucocorticoid action in bone. Ann N Y Acad Sci 2002;966:73–81.
6. Gordon CM, Zemel BS, Wren TA, et al. The Determinants of Peak Bone Mass. J Pediatr 2017;180:261–9.
7. Ji L, Lili S, Jing W, et al. Appearance concern and depression in adolescent girls with systemic lupus erythematous. Clin Rheumatol 2012;31:1671–5.
8. Knight A, Vickery M, Fiks AG, et al. The illness experience of youth with lupus/mixed connective tissue disease: a mixed methods analysis of patient and parent perspectives. Lupus 2016;25:1028–39.
9. Tektonidou MG, Lewandowski LB, Hu J, et al. Survival in adults and children with systemic lupus erythematosus: a systematic review and Bayesian meta-analysis of studies from 1950 to 2016. Ann Rheum Dis 2017;76:2009–16.
10. Beukelman T, Haynes K, Curtis JR, et al. Rates of malignancy associated with juvenile idiopathic arthritis and its treatment. Arthritis Rheum 2012;64:1263–71.
11. Roman MJ, Shanker BA, Davis A, et al. Prevalence and correlates of accelerated atherosclerosis in systemic lupus erythematosus. N Engl J Med 2003;349:2399–406.
12. White PH, Ardoin S. Transitioning Wisely: Improving the Connection From Pediatric to Adult Health Care. Arthritis Rheum 2016;68:789–94.
13. Ota S, Cron RQ, Schanberg LE, et al. Research priorities in pediatric rheumatology: The Childhood Arthritis and Rheumatology Research Alliance (CARRA) consensus. Pediatr Rheumatol Online J 2008;6:5.
14. Kimura Y, Grevich S, Beukelman T, et al. Pilot study comparing the Childhood Arthritis & Rheumatology Research Alliance (CARRA) systemic Juvenile

Idiopathic Arthritis Consensus Treatment Plans. Pediatr Rheumatol Online J 2017; 15:23.

15. Cooper JC, Rouster-Stevens K, Wright TB, et al. Pilot study comparing the childhood arthritis and rheumatology research alliance consensus treatment plans for induction therapy of juvenile proliferative lupus nephritis. Pediatr Rheumatol Online J 2018;16:65.

16. Prakken B, Albani S, Martini A. Juvenile idiopathic arthritis. Lancet 2011;377: 2138–49.

17. Kim KH, Kim DS. Juvenile idiopathic arthritis: Diagnosis and differential diagnosis. Korean J Pediatr 2010;53:931–5.

18. Thierry S, Fautrel B, Lemelle I, et al. Prevalence and incidence of juvenile idiopathic arthritis: a systematic review. Joint Bone Spine 2014;81:112–7.

19. Harrold LR, Salman C, Shoor S, et al. Incidence and prevalence of juvenile idiopathic arthritis among children in a managed care population, 1996-2009. J Rheumatol 2013;40:1218–25.

20. Petty RE, Southwood TR, Manners P, et al. International League of Associations for Rheumatology classification of juvenile idiopathic arthritis: second revision, Edmonton, 2001. J Rheumatol 2004;31:390–2.

21. Gowdie PJ, Tse SM. Juvenile idiopathic arthritis. Pediatr Clin North Am 2012;59: 301–27.

22. Martini A, Ravelli A, Avcin T, et al. Toward New Classification Criteria for Juvenile Idiopathic Arthritis: First Steps, Pediatric Rheumatology International Trials Organization International Consensus. J Rheumatol 2019;46:190–7.

23. Eng SWM, Aeschlimann FA, van Veenendaal M, et al. Patterns of joint involvement in juvenile idiopathic arthritis and prediction of disease course: A prospective study with multilayer non-negative matrix factorization. PLoS Med 2019;16: e1002750.

24. Bazso A, Consolaro A, Ruperto N, et al. Development and testing of reduced joint counts in juvenile idiopathic arthritis. J Rheumatol 2009;36:183–90.

25. Crayne CB, Beukelman T. Juvenile Idiopathic Arthritis: Oligoarthritis and Polyarthritis. Pediatr Clin North Am 2018;65:657–74.

26. Cabral DA, Petty RE, Fung M, et al. Persistent antinuclear antibodies in children without identifiable inflammatory rheumatic or autoimmune disease. Pediatrics 1992;89:441–4.

27. McGhee JL, Kickingbird LM, Jarvis JN. Clinical utility of antinuclear antibody tests in children. BMC Pediatr 2004;4:13.

28. Mehta J. Laboratory testing in pediatric rheumatology. Pediatr Clin North Am 2012;59:263–84.

29. Allen RC, Dewez P, Stuart L, et al. Antinuclear antibodies using HEp-2 cells in normal children and in children with common infections. J Paediatr Child Health 1991;27:39–42.

30. Hinks A, Marion MC, Cobb J, et al. Brief Report: The Genetic Profile of Rheumatoid Factor-Positive Polyarticular Juvenile Idiopathic Arthritis Resembles That of Adult Rheumatoid Arthritis. Arthritis Rheum 2018;70:957–62.

31. Smith JA. Testing for Rheumatological Diagnoses in Children. Eur Paediatr Rev 2009;3:30–4.

32. Angeles-Han ST, McCracken C, Yeh S, et al. Characteristics of a cohort of children with Juvenile Idiopathic Arthritis and JIA-associated Uveitis. Pediatr Rheumatol Online J 2015;13:19.

33. Hayworth JL, Turk MA, Nevskaya T, et al. The frequency of uveitis in patients with juvenile inflammatory rheumatic diseases. Joint Bone Spine 2019;86:685–90.

34. Cassidy J, Kivlin J, Lindsley C, et al. Ophthalmologic examinations in children with juvenile rheumatoid arthritis. Pediatrics 2006;117:1843–5.

35. Heiligenhaus A, Niewerth M, Ganser G, et al. German Uveitis in Childhood Study G. Prevalence and complications of uveitis in juvenile idiopathic arthritis in a population-based nation-wide study in Germany: suggested modification of the current screening guidelines. Rheumatology 2007;46:1015–9.

36. Lee JJY, Duffy CM, Guzman J, et al. Prospective Determination of the Incidence and Risk Factors of New-Onset Uveitis in Juvenile Idiopathic Arthritis: The Research in Arthritis in Canadian Children Emphasizing Outcomes Cohort. Arthritis Care Res 2019;71:1436–43.

37. Angeles-Han ST, Ringold S, Beukelman T, et al. 2019 American College of Rheumatology/Arthritis Foundation Guideline for the Screening, Monitoring, and Treatment of Juvenile Idiopathic Arthritis-Associated Uveitis. Arthritis Care Res 2019; 71:703–16.

38. Tay-Kearney ML, Schwam BL, Lowder C, et al. Clinical features and associated systemic diseases of HLA-B27 uveitis. Am J Ophthalmol 1996;121:47–56.

39. Sharma SM, Jackson D. Uveitis and spondyloarthropathies. Best Pract Res Clin Rheumatol 2017;31:846–62.

40. Giannini EH, Ruperto N, Ravelli A, et al. Preliminary definition of improvement in juvenile arthritis. Arthritis Rheum 1997;40:1202–9.

41. Consolaro A, Ruperto N, Bazso A, et al. Development and validation of a composite disease activity score for juvenile idiopathic arthritis. Arthritis Rheum 2009;61:658–66.

42. Horneff G, Becker I. Definition of improvement in juvenile idiopathic arthritis using the juvenile arthritis disease activity score. Rheumatology 2014;53:1229–34.

43. Wallace CA, Ruperto N, Giannini E, et al. Preliminary criteria for clinical remission for select categories of juvenile idiopathic arthritis. J Rheumatol 2004;31:2290–4.

44. Wallace CA, Huang B, Bandeira M, et al. Patterns of clinical remission in select categories of juvenile idiopathic arthritis. Arthritis Rheum 2005;52:3554–62.

45. Morgan EM, Munro JE, Horonjeff J, et al. Establishing an Updated Core Domain Set for Studies in Juvenile Idiopathic Arthritis: A Report from the OMERACT 2018 JIA Workshop. J Rheumatol 2019;46:1006–13.

46. Barut K, Adrovic A, Sahin S, et al. Prognosis, complications and treatment response in systemic juvenile idiopathic arthritis patients: A single-center experience. Int J Rheum Dis 2019;22:1661–9.

47. Simon S, Whiffen J, Shapiro F. Leg-length discrepancies in monoarticular and pauciarticular juvenile rheumatoid arthritis. J Bone Joint Surg Am 1981;63: 209–15.

48. Fellas A, Hawke F, Santos D, et al. Prevalence, presentation and treatment of lower limb pathologies in juvenile idiopathic arthritis: A narrative review. J Paediatr Child Health 2017;53:836–40.

49. Ozawa R, Inaba Y, Mori M, et al. Definitive differences in laboratory and radiological characteristics between two subtypes of juvenile idiopathic arthritis: systemic arthritis and polyarthritis. Mod Rheumatol 2012;22:558–64.

50. Stoll ML, Kau CH, Waite PD, et al. Temporomandibular joint arthritis in juvenile idiopathic arthritis, now what? Pediatr Rheumatol Online J 2018;16:32.

51. Glerup M, Stoustrup P, Matzen LH, et al. Longterm Outcomes of Temporomandibular Joints in Juvenile Idiopathic Arthritis: 17 Years of Followup of a Nordic Juvenile Idiopathic Arthritis Cohort. J Rheumatol 2019;47(5):730–8.

52. Hospach T, Maier J, Muller-Abt P, et al. Cervical spine involvement in patients with juvenile idiopathic arthritis - MRI follow-up study. Pediatr Rheumatol Online J 2014;12:9.

53. Ringold S, Weiss PF, Beukelman T, et al. 2013 update of the 2011 American College of Rheumatology recommendations for the treatment of juvenile idiopathic arthritis: recommendations for the medical therapy of children with systemic juvenile idiopathic arthritis and tuberculosis screening among children receiving biologic medications. Arthritis Rheum 2013;65:2499–512.

54. Ringold S, Angeles-Han ST, Beukelman T, et al. 2019 American College of Rheumatology/Arthritis Foundation Guideline for the Treatment of Juvenile Idiopathic Arthritis: Therapeutic Approaches for Non-Systemic Polyarthritis, Sacroiliitis, and Enthesitis. Arthritis Care Res 2019;71:717–34.

55. Giancane G, Muratore V, Marzetti V, et al. Disease activity and damage in juvenile idiopathic arthritis: methotrexate era versus biologic era. Arthritis Res Ther 2019; 21:168.

56. Huang BQT, Chen C, Zhang Y, et al. Timing matters: real-world effectiveness of early combination of biologic and conventional synthetic disease-modifying antirheumatic drugs for treating newly diagnosed polyarticular course juvenile idiopathic arthritis. RMD Open 2020;6:1–10.

57. Guzman J, Oen K, Loughin T. Predicting disease severity and remission in juvenile idiopathic arthritis: are we getting closer? Curr Opin Rheumatol 2019;31: 436–49.

58. Adib N, Davies K, Grahame R, et al. Joint hypermobility syndrome in childhood. A not so benign multisystem disorder? Rheumatology 2005;44:744–50.

59. Kumar B, Lenert P. Joint Hypermobility Syndrome: Recognizing a Commonly Overlooked Cause of Chronic Pain. Am J Med 2017;130:640–7.

60. Achar S, Yamanaka J. Apophysitis and Osteochondrosis: Common Causes of Pain in Growing Bones. Am Fam Physician 2019;99:610–8.

61. Gaitonde DY, Ericksen A, Robbins RC. Patellofemoral Pain Syndrome. Am Fam Physician 2019;99:88–94.

62. Do TT. Transient synovitis as a cause of painful limps in children. Curr Opin Pediatr 2000;12:48–51.

63. Boteanu AL, Sifuentes-Giraldo WA, Anton-Pages F, et al. Osteoid osteoma of the knee mimicking juvenile psoriatic arthritis. Reumatol Clin 2017;13:240–2.

64. Willimon SC, Busch MT, Perkins CA. Pigmented Villonodular Synovitis of the Knee: An Underappreciated Source of Pain in Children and Adolescents. J Pediatr Orthop 2018;38:e482–5.

65. Bouayed K, Cherqaoui A, Salam S, et al. Lipoma arborescens: A rare cause of bilateral pseudo-arthritis of the knee in children. Joint Bone Spine 2017;84: 639–40.

66. Boccuzzi E, Ferro VA, Cinicola B, et al. Uncommon Presentation of Childhood Leukemia in Emergency Department: The Usefulness of an Early Multidisciplinary Approach. Pediatr Emerg Care 2018. [Epub ahead of print].

67. Li SC. Scleroderma in Children and Adolescents: Localized Scleroderma and Systemic Sclerosis. Pediatr Clin North Am 2018;65:757–81.

68. Herrick AL, Ennis H, Bhushan M, et al. Clinical features of childhood localized scleroderma in an incidence cohort. Rheumatology 2011;50:1865–8.

69. Zulian F, Balzarin M, Birolo C. Recent advances in the management of juvenile systemic sclerosis. Expert Rev Clin Immunol 2017;13:361–9.

70. Martini G, Vittadello F, Kasapcopur O, et al. Factors affecting survival in juvenile systemic sclerosis. Rheumatology 2009;48:119–22.

71. Foeldvari I, Nihtyanova SI, Wierk A, et al. Characteristics of patients with juvenile onset systemic sclerosis in an adult single-center cohort. J Rheumatol 2010;37: 2422–6.
72. Torok KS. Pediatric scleroderma: systemic or localized forms. Pediatr Clin North Am 2012;59:381–405.
73. Peterson LS, Nelson AM, Su WP, et al. The epidemiology of morphea (localized scleroderma) in Olmsted County 1960-1993. J Rheumatol 1997;24:73–80.
74. Zulian F, Vallongo C, Woo P, et al. Localized scleroderma in childhood is not just a skin disease. Arthritis Rheum 2005;52:2873–81.
75. Lythgoe H, Almeida B, Bennett J, et al. Multi-centre national audit of juvenile lo-calised scleroderma: describing current UK practice in disease assessment and management. Pediatr Rheumatol Online J 2018;16:80.
76. Wu EY, Li SC, Torok KS, et al. Baseline Description of the Juvenile Localized Scleroderma Subgroup From the Childhood Arthritis and Rheumatology Research Alliance Legacy Registry. ACR Open Rheumatol 2019;1:119–24.
77. Torok KS, Li SC, Jacobe HM, et al. Immunopathogenesis of Pediatric Localized Scleroderma. Front Immunol 2019;10:908.
78. Saracino AM, Denton CP, Orteu CH. The molecular pathogenesis of morphoea: from genetics to future treatment targets. Br J Dermatol 2017;177:34–46.
79. Laxer RM, Zulian F. Localized scleroderma. Curr Opin Rheumatol 2006;18: 606–13.
80. Zulian F, Athreya BH, Laxer R, et al. Juvenile localized scleroderma: clinical and epidemiological features in 750 children. An international study. Rheumatology 2006;45:614–20.
81. Zulian F. Scleroderma in children. Best Pract Res Clin Rheumatol 2017;31: 576–95.
82. Vancheeswaran R, Black CM, David J, et al. Childhood-onset scleroderma: is it different from adult-onset disease. Arthritis Rheum 1996;39:1041–9.
83. Porter AME, Fritzler MJ, Brown R, et al. Autoantibody Testing in Pediatric Local-ized Scleroderma (LS) [abstract]. Arthritis Rheum 2018;70.
84. Chiu YE, Vora S, Kwon EK, et al. A significant proportion of children with morphea en coup de sabre and Parry-Romberg syndrome have neuroimaging findings. Pediatr Dermatol 2012;29:738–48.
85. Fledelius HC, Danielsen PL, Ullman S. Ophthalmic findings in linear scleroderma manifesting as facial en coup de sabre. Eye (Lond) 2018;32:1688–96.
86. Horberg M, Lauesen SR, Daugaard-Jensen J, et al. Linear scleroderma en coup de sabre including abnormal dental development. Eur Arch Paediatr Dent 2015; 16:227–31.
87. Constantin T, Foeldvari I, Pain CE, et al. Development of minimum standards of care for juvenile localized scleroderma. Eur J Pediatr 2018;177:961–77.
88. Kelsey CE, Torok KS. The Localized Scleroderma Cutaneous Assessment Tool: responsiveness to change in a pediatric clinical population. J Am Acad Dermatol 2013;69:214–20.
89. Lis-Swiety A, Janicka I, Skrzypek-Salamon A, et al. A systematic review of tools for determining activity of localized scleroderma in paediatric and adult patients. J Eur Acad Dermatol Venereol 2017;31:30–7.
90. Zulian F, Culpo R, Sperotto F, et al. Consensus-based recommendations for the management of juvenile localised scleroderma. Ann Rheum Dis 2019;78: 1019–24.

91. Martini G, Ramanan AV, Falcini F, et al. Successful treatment of severe or methotrexate-resistant juvenile localized scleroderma with mycophenolate mofetil. Rheumatology 2009;48:1410–3.
92. Mertens JS, Marsman D, van de Kerkhof PC, et al. Use of Mycophenolate Mofetil in Patients with Severe Localized Scleroderma Resistant or Intolerant to Methotrexate. Acta Derm Venereol 2016;96:510–3.
93. Li SC, Torok KS, Rabinovich CE, et al. Initial Results from a Pilot Comparative Effectiveness Study of Three Methotrexate-Based Consensus Treatment Plans for Juvenile Localized Scleroderma. J Rheumatol 2020;47(8):1242–52.
94. Kurzinski KL, Zigler CK, Torok KS. Prediction of disease relapse in a cohort of paediatric patients with localized scleroderma. Br J Dermatol 2019;180:1183–9.
95. Hawley DP, Baildam EM, Amin TS, et al. Access to care for children and young people diagnosed with localized scleroderma or juvenile SSc in the UK. Rheumatology 2012;51:1235–9.

Overview of Pediatric Rheumatology: Part Two

Heather Benham, DNP, APRN, CPNP-PC[a],*, Tracey B. Wright, MD[b]

KEYWORDS

- Systemic lupus erythematosus • Juvenile dermatomyositis • Vasculitis
- Autoinflammatory syndromes

KEY POINTS

- When systemic lupus erythematosus presents in childhood, there is high risk for major organ involvement, particularly nephritis, and accrual of irreversible damage.
- Children with juvenile dermatomyositis have increased risk for calcinosis compared with those with adult-onset disease.
- Kawasaki disease is a self-limited vasculitis unique to childhood.
- A broad spectrum of autoinflammatory syndromes can present in childhood.

BRIEF INTRODUCTION

Part two of this review on pediatric rheumatic diseases focuses on systemic lupus erythematosus, juvenile dermatomyositis and vasculitis, with particular emphasis on how the presentations, manifestations and prognoses of these diseases differ from the adult population. In addition, there is a brief review of some of the most common autoinflammatory syndromes in childhood.

SYSTEMIC LUPUS ERYTHEMATOSUS

Approximately 20% of systemic lupus erythematosus (SLE) cases are diagnosed before age of 16. The estimated incidence is 0.3 to 0.9 per 100, 000 children-years.[1] Several studies comparing the clinical features of adult and pediatric lupus highlight children commonly manifest major organ involvement and more frequently accrue damage than adults.[2] Children have also been shown to have higher Systemic Lupus Erythematosus Disease Activity Index (SLEDAI) scores at presentation in children when compared with adults and have been found in addition and to have increased renal disease activity over time[3]

[a] Pediatric Rheaumtology, Scottish Rite Hospital, 2222 Welborn Street, Dallas, TX 75219, USA;
[b] Division of Rheumatology, Department of Pediatrics, UT Southwestern Medical Center, 5323 Harry Hines Boulevard, MC 9063, Dallas, TX 75390, USA
* Corresponding author.
E-mail address: heather.benham@tsrh.org

Physician Assist Clin 6 (2021) 193–207
https://doi.org/10.1016/j.cpha.2020.09.003
2405-7991/21/© 2020 Elsevier Inc. All rights reserved.

Clinical features in childhood lupus differ in specific ways from those in adult-onset disease. Mucocutaneous manifestations are quite common in children, apart from the occurrence of discoid rash without systemic features.[4] Arthritis occurs frequently though the majority of patients rarely develop chronic arthritis as is seen in juvenile idiopathic arthritis.[5] Autoimmune hemolytic anemia is more prevalent and severe in children.[6] Although thrombotic thrombocytopenic purpura in childhood is most frequently associated with SLE,[7] macrophage activation syndrome is a rare but severe hematologic and multi-organ manifestation.[8] Lupus nephritis is more prevalent occurring in 40% to 70% of pediatric SLE and is a common cause of morbidity and mortality.[9] Myocardial disease may occur more often than previously realized with a greater prevalence of pericarditis and myocarditis compared with adults.[10] Neuropsychiatric disease may occur at presentation or several years after diagnosis.[11] Chorea is a rare neuropsychiatric manifestation occurring more frequently in children.[12] Similar to adults, the SLEDAI and systemic lupus international collaborating clinics (SLICC) Damage Index are the most frequently used tools to assess disease activity and damage. The SLICC Damage Index, however, does not account for features unique to children including growth issues and delay in onset of menstruation.[13]

Several quality indicators have been identified to guide disease management in pediatric SLE.[14] Special attention to the vaccination status of children is important as patients are especially susceptible to severe infection, an important cause of mortality.[15] Monitoring bone health is essential, as patients who develop SLE in childhood have a much greater risk of steroid-related damage (ie, osteoporosis with fracture, AVN, cataracts, and diabetes) compared with adult-onset disease, notably when there is longer disease duration.[16] Recent studies confirm adults who were diagnosed with lupus in childhood developed damage, had reduced health related quality of life and continued to need ongoing therapy.[17]

Medications are selected according to clinical manifestations in a manner similar to the treatment approach for adults with SLE. Further study of the approach needed for pediatric SLE is described as an urgent gap in knowledge as there is a need to improve understanding of pediatric drug dosing and length of therapy.[18] Childhood and arthritis rheumatology alliance (CARRA) has published Consensus Treatment Plans providing guidance in the management of proliferative nephritis.[19,20] Biologic therapy has been studied and approved in pediatric SLE.[21]

JUVENILE DERMATOMYOSITIS

Juvenile dermatomyositis (JDM), although a rare condition, is the most common idiopathic inflammatory myopathy in childhood.[22,23] Estimated annual incidence is 1.9 to 3.2 cases per million[24,25] with typical median age of onset ranging from 5.7 to 7.7 years.[26–29] The primary manifestations are proximal muscle weakness and prototypic typical rashes, however, presentation can be variable.[30] Although the exact etiology of JDM is still unclear, there are known genetic and environmental factors, including sun exposure, which likely contribute to immune dysfunction.[31,32] Both the innate and adaptive immune systems contribute to pathogenesis.[22,33]

The current diagnostic criteria used in clinical practice were developed by Bohan and Peter[34] in 1975 and include 5 components: (1) muscle weakness, (2) muscle biopsy findings, (3) elevated skeletal muscle enzymes, (4) electromyography (EMG) changes, and (5) dermatologic features. However, new data-driven EULAR/ACR criteria have recently been published using defined clinical and laboratory parameters.[35] Systematic review of these components, with or without muscle biopsy results, provides a score corresponding to the probability of having an idiopathic inflammatory myopathy.

Children with JDM typically present with symmetric muscle weakness, most often in the proximal muscle groups.[22,36] and may have dysphonia and/or dysphagia due to weakness of the muscles of the palate and around the pharynx.[36,37] Typical rashes include heliotrope (purplish/violaceous discoloration around the eyes), Gottron papules and periungual erythema with capillaropathy.[37–39] Cutaneous vasculitis and ulcerations may be associated with a more persistent and severe disease course[40] and occur in more than 20% of children at presentation in several cohorts.[26,38]

Arthritis also occurs[30,36] with a recent study revealing this manifestation in more than 40% of patients with JDM during the course of their disease.[37] Gastrointestinal manifestations can be mild including abdominal pain and reflux, however, vasculopathy can result in bleeding, ulceration or perforation.[31,39] Pulmonary involvement can include respiratory muscle weakness, aspiration pneumonia and interstitial lung disease (ILD).[41] Children with JDM can also develop dystrophic calcifications (**Figs. 1** and **2**), which, if extensive, can impact joint range of motion and tissue integrity.[42,43]

Diagnosis is usually established based on history (weakness, fatigue, endurance issues), physical findings, and elevated serum muscle esnzymes.[23,26,38] MRI of the pelvis reveals increased signal intensity within the affected muscles on T2-weighted

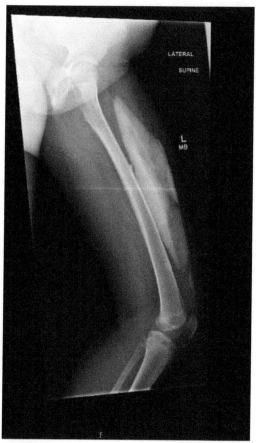

Fig. 1. Dystrophic calcifications in the anterior thigh of a patient with JDM.

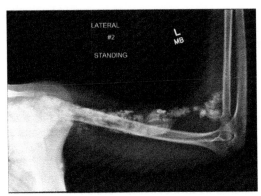

Fig. 2. Dystrophic calcifications in the upper extremity and anterior chest wall of a patient with JDM.

images, perimuscular edema, and changes to the subcutaneous fat.[44] Many centers use muscle biopsy to confirm the diagnosis; classic findings include perifasicular atrophy, perivascular inflammation, muscle fiber degeneration/regeneration, and tubuloreticular inclusion bodies.[31] Although EMG is included in the historical diagnostic criteria, this is used less often due to risk for nondiagnostic results[27] and is not well tolerated by children.

Similar to dermatomyositis in adults, myositis-specific antibodies and myositis-associated antibodies help delineate clinical phenotypes and determine risk for certain disease manifestations/complications.[45,46] There are differences in the frequencies of these antibodies in JDM versus adult-onset disease, likely leading to variations in observed clinical phenotypes.[45] Certainly, while JDM patients have increased incidence of calcinosis compared with adults, they have a lower incidence of ILD and no clear risk for malignancy.[23,46] When establishing a diagnosis of JDM, it is important to consider atypical presentations, including rash without significant muscle involvement (amyopathic disease), as well as other etiologies for muscle weakness or myositis, including dystrophies, infections, endocrine disorders or metabolic diseases.[23]

Treatment of JDM typically includes steroids, often a combination of oral steroids and intravenous (IV) methylprednisolone pulses, IV immunoglobulin (IVIG), methotrexate, and mycophenolate.[47] Refractory disease is frequently treated with IVIG, while there have also been trials looking at the use of various biologic therapies.[47] Consensus-based recommendations for the management of JDM have recently been published.[48] In addition, there are multiple measures, which can be used to assess disease activity and response to therapy.[49,50]

Disease course can be monocyclic, polycyclic or persistent/recalcitrant.[29,40,51] Flares are often associated with sun exposure and infection.[52] Despite ongoing efforts toward earlier recognition and more standardized treatment regimens, many JDM patients have persistently active disease and incur long-term damage including cutaneous scar, muscle atrophy and dysfunction, lipodystrophy and joint contractures.[53]

VASCULITIS

The classification criteria for vasculitis in childhood are adapted from classification criteria used in adults.[54,55]

Antineutrophil Cytoplasmic Antibody–Associated Vasculitis

Small to medium size vessel vasculitis is rare in childhood. A detailed review of anti-neutrophil cytoplasmic antibody–associated vasculitis (AAV) is provided elsewhere in this journal and many clinical manifestations are similar between children and adults though some clinical features are distinct in childhood. AAV is more common in female individuals and tends to occur in late childhood into adolescence.[56] The estimated incidence of granulomatosus with polyangiitis in children is 0.28 to 0.64 per 100,000 per year.[57] Disease of the upper and lower respiratory tracts are common presenting features in children.[58] Of the upper respiratory tract manifestations that occur, sub-glottic stenosis is much more common in children.[59] A Pediatric Vasculitis Activity Score has been developed to monitor disease activity.[60] The approach to treatment of pediatric AAV is based on clinical trials performed in adults underscoring the need for further study in children.[61]

Kawasaki Disease

Kawasaki disease (KD) is a self-limited vasculitis unique to childhood characterized by fever, conjunctivitis (**Fig. 3**), cervical adenopathy, mucosal changes (**Fig. 4**), rash, and erythema and edema of the hands and feet in the acute phase.[62] The major complication of KD is the development of coronary artery aneurysms when there is a delay in diagnosis and treatment. KD tends to occur in early childhood with most children developing the disease before 5 years of age and is slightly more common in boys.[63] Because KD has the highest incidence in patients of Asian race, current studies are focused on understanding genetic susceptibility and have revealed genes associated with increased predisposition to KD.[63] While an infectious trigger is suspected, a specific pathogen has not been identified.

The American Heart Association has established diagnostic criteria.[62] KD is characterized by 3 clinical phases if untreated. The acute febrile phase may last 10 to 14 days. Patients present in this phase with sudden onset of fever followed by conjunctivitis, enlarged cervical lymph nodes, mucositis, rash, and hand and foot erythema and edema. Patients are quite irritable. The fever is characteristically high, approximately 40° Celsius. The conjunctivitis is characterized by limbic sparing and lack of exudate (see **Fig. 3**). The mucositis is characterized by a "strawberry tongue" and swollen, cracked lips (see **Fig. 4**). The rash is nonspecific and typically begins on the trunk. Adenitis usually manifests as an enlarged, single cervical node. Beyond laboratory evidence of systemic inflammation, there is marked thrombocytosis up to 1,000,000/mm^3. Without treatment, these clinical manifestations will resolve by the

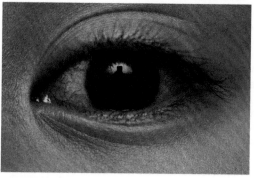

Fig. 3. Conjunctivitis associated with KD.

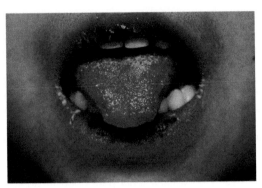

Fig. 4. Mucosal changes associated with KD.

end of this phase.[62] In the subacute phase, which may last 2 to 4 weeks, patients develop a characteristic desquamation of the finger and toes. Coronary artery aneurysms develop during this phase. The convalescent phase may last for months or longer and is the phase in which patients are asymptomatic and the blood vessels are healing.[62]

Because patients may not exhibit all clinical manifestations of KD, it is imperative to maintain a high level of suspicion in young children with persistent fever. Approximately a quarter of untreated KD will result in coronary artery aneurysms and thus the echocardiogram is an essential tool in the evaluation of these patients.[62] Most coronary artery changes can be detected on the initial echocardiogram underscoring the need for early detection and treatment.[64] Thrombosis or rupture of coronary artery aneurysms may ultimately result in myocardial infarction or death, with the highest risk in those with giant aneurysms.[63] The American Heart Association recommends patients receive aspirin and IVIG within the first 10 days of the start of symptoms.[62] Historically, primary treatment has consisted of anti-inflammatory doses of aspirin during the acute febrile phase followed by antiplatelet doses of aspirin until laboratory studies normalize. IVIG has been shown to be remarkably effective in reducing the occurrence of coronary artery aneurysms and should be given within the first 10 days of symptoms for maximal effectiveness.[65] Recent studies demonstrate the effectiveness of steroids and biologic therapy in halting the progression of coronary artery aneurysms.[66]

Henoch Schonlein Purpura

Henoch Schonlein purpura, sometimes also referred to as "IgA vasculitis," is a common small vessel vasculitis in childhood that rarely occurs in adults. It affects patients between the ages of 3 to 15 and is slightly more common in boys than girls with an estimated incidence of 9 to 86 per 100,000 with some variation by race/ethnicity and socioeconomic status.[67] There are multiple theories regarding pathogenesis including strep as a possible trigger.[68] The classic pathologic lesion is leukocytoclastic vasculitis with IgA deposition detected in skin and renal biopsies.[69] Palpable purpura, the most common clinical feature, is most noticeable on dependent areas including the buttocks and lower extremities[55] (**Fig. 5**). Subcutaneous edema occurs periorbitally, over the top of the hands and feet, and in the scrotum. Arthritis and arthralgias are transient, commonly affecting large joints manifested by "periarticular swelling" and joint pain.[70] Gastrointestinal disease may occur in 51% to 74% of patients developing 1 to 4 weeks after the rash appears.[71] Patients have risk of intestinal vasculitis

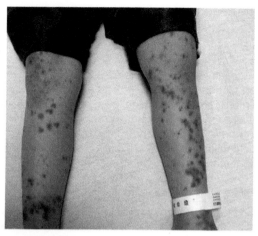

Fig. 5. Palpable purpura on the lower extremities.

with subsequent small bowel intussusception. Gangrene and perforation are less common but are a medical emergency.[71] Glomerulonephritis may present with microscopic hematuria and mild proteinuria. Any manifestation suggesting severe renal disease warrants further evaluation with renal biopsy as there is a risk of progression to end stage renal disease. Presence of nephrotic syndrome and crescents on biopsy are amongst the risk factors associated with poor outcomes.[72] Because renal disease may occur later, it is imperative to follow blood pressures and urinalyses over time for approximately 6 months to assess for future development of renal disease.[73] Treatment is primarily supportive including nonsteroidal anti-inflammatory drugs (NSAIDs) for pain and joint symptoms. The use of steroids is controversial but may be indicated for the treatment of severe gastrointestinal disease.[74,75]

PERIODIC FEVERS AND AUTOINFLAMMATORY SYNDROMES

Autoinflammatory syndromes are a group of disorders characterized by dysregulation of the innate immune system with recurrent fevers as the primary clinical hallmark. Most hereditary autoinflammatory syndromes are characterized by monogenic defects. As an in-depth description of autoinflammatory diseases is beyond the scope of this review, only the most common disorders are discussed. The reader is directed to several existing comprehensive reviews describing the full spectrum of the known autoinflammatory syndromes.[76,77]

Familial Mediterranean Fever

Familial Mediterranean fever arises from an autosomal recessive mutation in the MEFV "locus" on chromosome 16 p.[78] Disease may begin during childhood or adolescence and is characterized by recurrent episodes of symptoms typically lasting 2 to 3 days. Clinical manifestations include fever, abdominal pain that may be severe, arthralgia/arthritis, and rash, classically described as "an erysipeloid erythematous rash" predominantly on the lower extremities.[79] Laboratory evidence of systemic inflammation is evident during periods of clinical symptoms. Colchicine is the mainstay of therapy in the majority of patients.[80] Anti-interleukin (IL)-1 therapy is increasingly used in patients who do not respond to colchicine.[81]

Tumor Necrosis Factor Receptor–Associated Periodic Syndrome

Tumor necrosis factor receptor–associated periodic syndrome (TRAPS) results from a variants in in the TNFRSFIA gene. Although many mutations are inherited in an autosomal dominant, cases of genetic heterogeneity lead to varied presentations there is some genetic heterogeneity resulting in varied presentations.[82] Patients experience recurrent episodes of longer duration lasting 1 to 4 weeks at a time. Clinical features may be variable but most commonly include fever, rash, predominantly on the trunk or extremities, abdominal pain, eye symptoms including periorbital edema or conjunctivitis, and arthralgia/arthritis.[83] Laboratory studies reveal systemic inflammation. Etanercept is commonly used as there is less experience with other anti–tumor necrosis factor (TNF) therapies.[84] Anti-IL-1 therapy is effective.[85]

Cryopyrin-Associated Periodic Fever Syndromes

Cryopyrin-associated periodic fever syndromes (CAPS) encompasses 3 syndromes caused by missense mutations in the NLRP3 gene generally inherited in an autosomal dominant pattern though sporadic cases may occur. CAPS are characterized by fever, rash, and joint symptoms: Familial Cold Autoinflammatory Syndrome (FCAS), Muckle-Wells Syndrome (MWS), and Neonatal-Onset Multisystem Inflammatory Disease (NOMID). FCAS is characterized by short, self-limited episodes of fever, rash, and arthralgia triggered by cold exposure.[86] Patients may also experience conjunctivitis, myalgias, and fatigue. These patients typically present in infancy. Constellation of symptoms may last less than 24 hours. In MWS, patients experience fever, rash, arthralgia/arthritis, conjunctivitis though fever may not always be present. Sensorineural hearing loss may occur in most patients. There is risk of future development of amyloidosis.[87] NOMID is the most severe phenotype with rash, joint symptoms and chronic aseptic meningitis. Symptoms occur at birth or in early infancy. Joint manifestations may be severe with marked bony hypertrophy and severe abnormalities on radiograph, including epiphyseal enlargement with abnormal ossification. Patients may experience various neurologic abnormalities including aseptic meningitis, uveitis, optic disc edema that may progress to blindness, and progressive hearing loss from chronic cochlear inflammation. Clinical manifestations are frequently severely disabling.[88] The mutations in CAPS results in overproduction of the proinflammatory cytokine IL-1β. As such, therapies targeting the IL 1 pathway have been revolutionary to the treatment of these patients.[88]

Chronic Recurrence Multifocal Osteomyelitis

Chronic recurrence multifocal osteomyelitis (CRMO) is an autoinflammatory disease characterized by inflammatory bone lesions not attributed to infection. CRMO may occur in isolation or in association with a variety of inflammatory diseases including inflammatory bowel disease.[89] Disease is more common in female individuals and tends to occur in middle childhood.[90] No specific inciting factor causes the development of bone inflammation and cultures do not reveal infection. The Bristol diagnostic criteria were published in 2016 and there are recent international efforts to develop and validate new classification criteria.[91,92] Localized bone pain is the predominant clinical symptom and may be associated with swelling. Lesions occur in 1 or multiple locations with the clavicle, spine, pelvis, and metaphysis of the long bones as the most common sites.[91,93] Fever and arthritis may occur and some patients develop a pustular rash. Laboratory studies reveal systemic inflammation. Imaging is critical to define extent of disease including detection of asymptomatic lesions. MRI is an especially useful tool revealing bone marrow edema and changes in signal intensity.[94] A biopsy reveals chronic inflammation and is useful to exclude infection and malignancy.[90] NSAIDs are first-line treatment and may be effective in a large number of patients.[95] However, lack of response to NSAIDs and/or extensive disease warrants therapy escalation. TNF inhibitors have proven to be effective[96,97] and bisphosphonates have been used in refractory cases.[98] CARRA has developed consensus treatment plans to guide therapy and addressed use of NSAIDs, TNF inhibitors, and palmidronate.[99] Although disease may be self-limited in some, many experience a prolonged course with ongoing disease more than 5 years after diagnosis.[95]

Periodic Fever with Aphthous Stomatitis, Pharyngitis, and Adenitis

Periodic fever with aphthous stomatitis, pharyngitis, and adenitis (PFAPA) is the most common of the periodic fever syndromes and has a benign course. Children tend to present in early childhood, before age 5, with fever episodes up to 40° C occurring every 4 weeks. Fever episodes are frequently predictable and high fevers may occur for up to 3 to 4 days with laboratory evidence of systemic inflammation. Clinical manifestations include fatigue, malaise, oral ulcers, cervical adenitis, and pharyngitis without signs of an intercurrent infection. Patients are well in between fever episodes and grow normally.[100] Because PFAPA is a diagnosis of exclusion, other recurrent autoinflammatory syndromes must be considered in the evaluation. There are no definitive treatment guidelines. Patients may receive an "abortive" prednisone up to 2 mg/kg given as a single dose at the beginning of symptoms. Although a dose of prednisone may indeed stop the episode, subsequent occurrences tend to be more frequent.[100] There are anecdotal reports of improvement with cimetidine and colchicine.[101] Tonsillectomy and adenoidectomy may also result in remission though evidence is limited.[102] Fever episodes tend to resolve by late childhood.

SUMMARY

The care of children with rheumatic diseases is challenging given the impact of inflammatory conditions and their treatments on growth and development, functional abilities, self-image, self-efficacy, and family dynamics. Delay in recognition and appropriate referral results in a significant, negative impact on outcomes. Therefore, it is important for clinicians to recognize the presenting symptoms and physical manifestations of these diseases. This review highlighted the most common rheumatic diseases in childhood and how they differ from similar diseases presenting in adulthood. Because these conditions may be diagnostically challenging, even an index of suspicion should prompt a referral to a pediatric rheumatologist for further work-up and initiation of early, aggressive treatment if warranted.

DISCLOSURE

The authors have nothing to disclose.

REFERENCES

1. Kamphuis S, Silverman ED. Prevalence and burden of pediatric-onset systemic lupus erythematosus. Nat Rev Rheumatol 2010;6:538–46.

2. Mina R, Brunner HI. Pediatric lupus–are there differences in presentation, genetics, response to therapy, and damage accrual compared with adult lupus? Rheum Dis Clin North Am 2010;36:53–80, vii-viii.

3. Brunner HI, Gladman DD, Ibanez D, et al. Difference in disease features between childhood-onset and adult-onset systemic lupus erythematosus. Arthritis Rheum 2008;58:556–62.

4. Chottawornsak N, Rodsaward P, Suwannachote S, et al. Skin signs in juvenile- and adult-onset systemic lupus erythematosus: clues to different systemic involvement. Lupus 2018;27:2069–75.

5. Silva CA. Childhood-onset systemic lupus erythematosus: early disease manifestations that the paediatrician must know. Expert Rev Clin Immunol 2016;12:907–10.

6. Gormezano NW, Kern D, Pereira OL, et al. Autoimmune hemolytic anemia in systemic lupus erythematosus at diagnosis: differences between pediatric and adult patients. Lupus 2017;26:426–30.

7. Brunner HI, Freedman M, Silverman ED. Close relationship between systemic lupus erythematosus and thrombotic thrombocytopenic purpura in childhood. Arthritis Rheum 1999;42:2346–55.

8. Borgia RE, Gerstein M, Levy DM, et al. Features, treatment, and outcomes of macrophage activation syndrome in childhood-onset systemic lupus erythematosus. Arthritis Rheumatol 2018;70:616–24.

9. Hiraki LT, Feldman CH, Liu J, et al. Prevalence, incidence, and demographics of systemic lupus erythematosus and lupus nephritis from 2000 to 2004 among children in the US Medicaid beneficiary population. Arthritis Rheum 2012;64:2669–76.

10. Chang JC, Xiao R, Mercer-Rosa L, et al. Child-onset systemic lupus erythematosus is associated with a higher incidence of myopericardial manifestations compared to adult-onset disease. Lupus 2018;27:2146–54.

11. Sibbitt WL Jr, Brandt JR, Johnson CR, et al. The incidence and prevalence of neuropsychiatric syndromes in pediatric onset systemic lupus erythematosus. J Rheumatol 2002;29:1536–42.

12. Athanasopoulos E, Kalaitzidou I, Vlachaki G, et al. Chorea revealing systemic lupus erythematosus in a 13-year old boy: A case report and short review of the literature. Int Rev Immunol 2018;37:177–82.

13. Gutierrez-Suarez R, Ruperto N, Gastaldi R, et al. A proposal for a pediatric version of the Systemic Lupus International Collaborating Clinics/American College of Rheumatology Damage Index based on the analysis of 1,015 patients with juvenile-onset systemic lupus erythematosus. Arthritis Rheum 2006;54:2989–96.

14. Hollander MC, Sage JM, Greenler AJ, et al. International consensus for provisions of quality-driven care in childhood-onset systemic lupus erythematosus. Arthritis Care Res 2013;65:1416–23.

15. Bernatsky S, Boivin JF, Joseph L, et al. Mortality in systemic lupus erythematosus. Arthritis Rheum 2006;54:2550–7.

16. Heshin-Bekenstein M, Trupin L, Yelin E, et al. Longitudinal disease- and steroid-related damage among adults with childhood-onset systemic lupus erythematosus. Semin Arthritis Rheum 2019;49:267–72.

17. Groot N, Shaikhani D, Teng YKO, et al. Long-term clinical outcomes in a cohort of adults with childhood-onset systemic lupus erythematosus. Arthritis Rheumatol 2019;71:290–301.

18. Ardoin SP, Daly RP, Merzoug L, et al. Research priorities in childhood-onset lupus: results of a multidisciplinary prioritization exercise. Pediatr Rheumatol Online J 2019;17:32.

19. Mina R, von Scheven E, Ardoin SP, et al. Consensus treatment plans for induction therapy of newly diagnosed proliferative lupus nephritis in juvenile systemic lupus erythematosus. Arthritis Care Res 2012;64:375–83.

20. Cooper JC, Rouster-Stevens K, Wright TB, et al. Pilot study comparing the childhood arthritis and rheumatology research alliance consensus treatment plans for induction therapy of juvenile proliferative lupus nephritis. Pediatr Rheumatol Online J 2018;16:65.

21. Brunner HI, Abud-Mendoza C, Viola DI, et al. Efficacy and safety of intravenous belimumab in children with systemic lupus erythematosus [abstract]. Arthritis Rheum 2018;70:1340–1348.

22. Rider LG, Nistala K. The juvenile idiopathic inflammatory myopathies: pathogenesis, clinical and autoantibody phenotypes, and outcomes. J Intern Med 2016; 280:24–38.

23. Huber AM. Juvenile idiopathic inflammatory myopathies. Pediatr Clin North Am 2018;65:739–56.

24. Symmons DP, Sills JA, Davis SM. The incidence of juvenile dermatomyositis: results from a nation-wide study. Br J Rheumatol 1995;34:732–6.

25. Mendez EP, Lipton R, Ramsey-Goldman R, et al. US incidence of juvenile dermatomyositis, 1995-1998: results from the National Institute of Arthritis and Musculoskeletal and Skin Diseases Registry. Arthritis Rheum 2003;49:300–5.

26. McCann LJ, Juggins AD, Maillard SM, et al. The Juvenile Dermatomyositis National Registry and Repository (UK and Ireland)–clinical characteristics of children recruited within the first 5 yr. Rheumatology 2006;45:1255–60.

27. Robinson AB, Hoeltzel MF, Wahezi DM, et al. Clinical characteristics of children with juvenile dermatomyositis: the Childhood Arthritis and Rheumatology Research Alliance Registry. Arthritis Care Res 2014;66:404–10.

28. Sun C, Lee JH, Yang YH, et al. Juvenile dermatomyositis: a 20-year retrospective analysis of treatment and clinical outcomes. Pediatr Neonatol 2015;56:31–9.

29. Al-Mayouf SM, AlMutiari N, Muzaffer M, et al. Phenotypic characteristics and outcome of juvenile dermatomyositis in Arab children. Rheumatol Int 2017;37: 1513–7.

30. Quartier P, Gherardi RK. Juvenile dermatomyositis. Handb Clin Neurol 2013; 113:1457–63.

31. Feldman BM, Rider LG, Reed AM, et al. Juvenile dermatomyositis and other idiopathic inflammatory myopathies of childhood. Lancet 2008;371:2201–12.

32. Wedderburn LR, Rider LG. Juvenile dermatomyositis: new developments in pathogenesis, assessment and treatment. Best Pract Res Clin Rheumatol 2009;23:665–78.

33. Rayavarapu S, Coley W, Kinder TB, et al. Idiopathic inflammatory myopathies: pathogenic mechanisms of muscle weakness. Skelet Muscle 2013;3:13.

34. Bohan A, Peter JB. Polymyositis and dermatomyositis (first of two parts). N Engl J Med 1975;292:344–7.

35. Lundberg IE, Tjarnlund A, Bottai M, et al. 2017 European League Against Rheumatism/American College of Rheumatology Classification Criteria for Adult and Juvenile Idiopathic Inflammatory Myopathies and Their Major Subgroups. Arthritis Rheumatol 2017;69:2271–82.

36. Batthish M, Feldman BM. Juvenile dermatomyositis. Curr Rheumatol Rep 2011; 13:216–24.

37. Shah M, Mamyrova G, Targoff IN, et al. The clinical phenotypes of the juvenile idiopathic inflammatory myopathies. Medicine (Baltimore) 2013;92:25–41.

38. Gowdie PJ, Allen RC, Kornberg AJ, et al. Clinical features and disease course of patients with juvenile dermatomyositis. Int J Rheum Dis 2013;16:561–7.

39. Papadopoulou C, McCann LJ. The vasculopathy of juvenile dermatomyositis. Front Pediatr 2018;6:284.

40. Bowyer SL, Blane CE, Sullivan DB, et al. Childhood dermatomyositis: factors predicting functional outcome and development of dystrophic calcification. J Pediatr 1983;103:882–8.

41. Pouessel G, Deschildre A, Le Bourgeois M, et al. The lung is involved in juvenile dermatomyositis. Pediatr Pulmonol 2013;48:1016–25.

42. Saini I, Kalaivani M, Kabra SK. Calcinosis in juvenile dermatomyositis: frequency, risk factors and outcome. Rheumatol Int 2016;36:961–5.

43. Hoeltzel MF, Oberle EJ, Robinson AB, et al. The presentation, assessment, pathogenesis, and treatment of calcinosis in juvenile dermatomyositis. Curr Rheumatol Rep 2014;16:467.

44. Hernandez RJ, Sullivan DB, Chenevert TL, et al. MR imaging in children with dermatomyositis: musculoskeletal findings and correlation with clinical and laboratory findings. AJR Am J Roentgenol 1993;161:359–66.

45. Rider LG, Shah M, Mamyrova G, et al. The myositis autoantibody phenotypes of the juvenile idiopathic inflammatory myopathies. Medicine (Baltimore) 2013;92: 223–43.

46. Tansley SL, McHugh NJ, Wedderburn LR. Adult and juvenile dermatomyositis: are the distinct clinical features explained by our current understanding of serological subgroups and pathogenic mechanisms? Arthritis Res Ther 2013; 15:211.

47. Rider LG, Katz JD, Jones OY. Developments in the classification and treatment of the juvenile idiopathic inflammatory myopathies. Rheum Dis Clin North Am 2013;39:877–904.

48. Bellutti Enders F, Bader-Meunier B, Baildam E, et al. Consensus-based recommendations for the management of juvenile dermatomyositis. Ann Rheum Dis 2017;76:329–40.

49. Rider LG, Aggarwal R, Pistorio A, et al. 2016 American College of Rheumatology/European League Against Rheumatism Criteria for Minimal, Moderate, and Major Clinical Response in Juvenile Dermatomyositis: An International Myositis Assessment and Clinical Studies Group/Paediatric Rheumatology International Trials Organisation Collaborative Initiative. Ann Rheum Dis 2017;76: 782–91.

50. Rider LG, Werth VP, Huber AM, et al. Measures of adult and juvenile dermatomyositis, polymyositis, and inclusion body myositis: Physician and Patient/Parent Global Activity, Manual Muscle Testing (MMT), Health Assessment Questionnaire (HAQ)/Childhood Health Assessment Questionnaire (C-HAQ), Childhood Myositis Assessment Scale (CMAS), Myositis Disease Activity Assessment Tool (MDAAT), Disease Activity Score (DAS), Short Form 36 (SF-36), Child Health Questionnaire (CHQ), physician global damage, Myositis Damage Index (MDI), Quantitative Muscle Testing (QMT), Myositis Functional Index-2 (FI-2), Myositis Activities Profile (MAP), Inclusion Body Myositis Functional Rating Scale (IBMFRS), Cutaneous Dermatomyositis Disease Area and Severity Index (CDASI), Cutaneous Assessment Tool (CAT), Dermatomyositis Skin Severity Index (DSSI), Skindex, and Dermatology Life Quality Index (DLQI). Arthritis Care Res 2011;63(Suppl 11):S118–57.

51. Spencer CH, Hanson V, Singsen BH, et al. Course of treated juvenile dermatomyositis. J Pediatr 1984;105:399–408.

52. Mamyrova G, Rider LG, Ehrlich A, et al. Environmental factors associated with disease flare in juvenile and adult dermatomyositis. Rheumatology 2017;56: 1342–7.
53. Ravelli A, Trail L, Ferrari C, et al. Long-term outcome and prognostic factors of juvenile dermatomyositis: a multinational, multicenter study of 490 patients. Arthritis Care Res 2010;62:63–72.
54. Ruperto N, Ozen S, Pistorio A, et al. EULAR/PRINTO/PRES criteria for Henoch-Schonlein purpura, childhood polyarteritis nodosa, childhood Wegener granulomatosis and childhood Takayasu arteritis: Ankara 2008. Part I: Overall methodology and clinical characterisation. Ann Rheum Dis 2010;69:790–7.
55. Ozen S, Pistorio A, Iusan SM, et al. EULAR/PRINTO/PRES criteria for Henoch-Schonlein purpura, childhood polyarteritis nodosa, childhood Wegener granulomatosis and childhood Takayasu arteritis: Ankara 2008. Part II: Final classification criteria. Ann Rheum Dis 2010;69:798–806.
56. Cabral DA, Canter DL, Muscal E, et al. Comparing presenting clinical features in 48 children with microscopic polyangiitis to 183 children who have granulomatosis with polyangiitis (Wegener's): An ARChiVe cohort study. Arthritis Rheumatol 2016;68:2514–26.
57. Grisaru S, Yuen GW, Miettunen PM, et al. Incidence of Wegener's granulomatosis in children. J Rheumatol 2010;37:440–2.
58. Cabral DA, Uribe AG, Benseler S, et al. Classification, presentation, and initial treatment of Wegener's granulomatosis in childhood. Arthritis Rheum 2009;60: 3413–24.
59. Rottem M, Fauci AS, Hallahan CW, et al. Wegener granulomatosis in children and adolescents: clinical presentation and outcome. J Pediatr 1993;122:26–31.
60. Dolezalova P, Price-Kuehne FE, Ozen S, et al. Disease activity assessment in childhood vasculitis: development and preliminary validation of the Paediatric Vasculitis Activity Score (PVAS). Ann Rheum Dis 2013;72:1628–33.
61. Westwell-Roper C, Lubieniecka JM, Brown KL, et al. Clinical practice variation and need for pediatric-specific treatment guidelines among rheumatologists caring for children with ANCA-associated vasculitis: an international clinician survey. Pediatr Rheumatol Online J 2017;15:61.
62. Newburger JW, Takahashi M, Gerber MA, et al. Diagnosis, treatment, and long-term management of Kawasaki disease: a statement for health professionals from the Committee on Rheumatic Fever, Endocarditis, and Kawasaki Disease, Council on Cardiovascular Disease in the Young, American Heart Association. Pediatrics 2004;114:1708–33.
63. McCrindle BW, Rowley AH, Newburger JW, et al. Diagnosis, treatment, and long-term management of Kawasaki Disease: a scientific statement for health professionals from the American Heart Association. Circulation 2017;135: e927–99.
64. Dominguez SR, Anderson MS, El-Adawy M, et al. Preventing coronary artery abnormalities: a need for earlier diagnosis and treatment of Kawasaki disease. Pediatr Infect Dis J 2012;31:1217–20.
65. Newburger JW, Takahashi M, Burns JC, et al. The treatment of Kawasaki syndrome with intravenous gamma globulin. N Engl J Med 1986;315:341–7.
66. Dionne A, Burns JC, Dahdah N, et al. Treatment intensification in patients with Kawasaki Disease and coronary aneurysm at diagnosis. Pediatrics 2019;143.
67. Farley TA, Gillespie S, Rasoulpour M, et al. Epidemiology of a cluster of Henoch-Schonlein purpura. Am J Dis Child 1989;143:798–803.

68. Masuda M, Nakanishi K, Yoshizawa N, et al. Group A streptococcal antigen in the glomeruli of children with Henoch-Schonlein nephritis. Am J Kidney Dis 2003;41:366–70.

69. Shin JI, Kim JH, Lee JS. The diagnostic value of IgA deposition in Henoch-Schonlein purpura. Pediatr Dermatol 2008;25:140–1 [author reply: 1].

70. Oni L, Sampath S. Childhood IgA vasculitis (Henoch Schonlein Purpura)-advances and knowledge gaps. Front Pediatr 2019;7:257.

71. Ebert EC. Gastrointestinal manifestations of Henoch-Schonlein Purpura. Dig Dis Sci 2008;53:2011–9.

72. Shi D, Chan H, Yang X, et al. Risk factors associated with IgA vasculitis with nephritis (Henoch-Schonlein purpura nephritis) progressing to unfavorable outcomes: A meta-analysis. PLoS One 2019;14:e0223218.

73. Narchi H. Risk of long term renal impairment and duration of follow up recommended for Henoch-Schonlein purpura with normal or minimal urinary findings: a systematic review. Arch Dis Child 2005;90:916–20.

74. Weiss PF, Feinstein JA, Luan X, et al. Effects of corticosteroid on Henoch-Schonlein purpura: a systematic review. Pediatrics 2007;120:1079–87.

75. Weiss PF, Klink AJ, Localio R, et al. Corticosteroids may improve clinical outcomes during hospitalization for Henoch-Schonlein purpura. Pediatrics 2010; 126:674–81.

76. Masters SL, Simon A, Aksentijevich I, et al. Horror autoinflammaticus: the molecular pathophysiology of autoinflammatory disease (*). Annu Rev Immunol 2009; 27:621–68.

77. de Jesus AA, Canna SW, Liu Y, et al. Molecular mechanisms in genetically defined autoinflammatory diseases: disorders of amplified danger signaling. Annu Rev Immunol 2015;33:823–74.

78. Ancient missense mutations in a new member of the RoRet gene family are likely to cause familial Mediterranean fever. The International FMF Consortium. Cell 1997;90:797–807.

79. Majeed HA, Rawashdeh M, el-Shanti H, et al. Familial Mediterranean fever in children: the expanded clinical profile. QJM 1999;92:309–18.

80. Ozen S, Demirkaya E, Erer B, et al. EULAR recommendations for the management of familial Mediterranean fever. Ann Rheum Dis 2016;75:644–51.

81. Kohler BM, Lorenz HM, Blank N. IL1-blocking therapy in colchicine-resistant familial Mediterranean fever. Eur J Rheumatol 2018;5:230–4.

82. Aksentijevich I, Galon J, Soares M, et al. The tumor-necrosis-factor receptor-associated periodic syndrome: new mutations in TNFRSF1A, ancestral origins, genotype-phenotype studies, and evidence for further genetic heterogeneity of periodic fevers. Am J Hum Genet 2001;69:301–14.

83. Lachmann HJ, Papa R, Gerhold K, et al. The phenotype of TNF receptor-associated autoinflammatory syndrome (TRAPS) at presentation: a series of 158 cases from the Eurofever/EUROTRAPS international registry. Ann Rheum Dis 2014;73:2160–7.

84. Bulua AC, Mogul DB, Aksentijevich I, et al. Efficacy of etanercept in the tumor necrosis factor receptor-associated periodic syndrome: a prospective, open-label, dose-escalation study. Arthritis Rheum 2012;64:908–13.

85. Gattorno M, Pelagatti MA, Meini A, et al. Persistent efficacy of anakinra in patients with tumor necrosis factor receptor-associated periodic syndrome. Arthritis Rheum 2008;58:1516–20.

86. Gattorno M, Hofer M, Federici S, et al. Classification criteria for autoinflammatory recurrent fevers. Ann Rheum Dis 2019;78:1025–32.

87. Hawkins PN, Lachmann HJ, Aganna E, et al. Spectrum of clinical features in Muckle-Wells syndrome and response to anakinra. Arthritis Rheum 2004;50: 607–12.
88. Goldbach-Mansky R, Dailey NJ, Canna SW, et al. Neonatal-onset multisystem inflammatory disease responsive to interleukin-1beta inhibition. N Engl J Med 2006;355:581–92.
89. Bousvaros A, Marcon M, Treem W, et al. Chronic recurrent multifocal osteomyelitis associated with chronic inflammatory bowel disease in children. Dig Dis Sci 1999;44:2500–7.
90. King SM, Laxer RM, Manson D, et al. Chronic recurrent multifocal osteomyelitis: a noninfectious inflammatory process. Pediatr Infect Dis J 1987;6:907–11.
91. Roderick MR, Shah R, Rogers V, et al. Chronic recurrent multifocal osteomyelitis (CRMO) - advancing the diagnosis. Pediatr Rheumatol Online J 2016;14:47.
92. Oliver M, Wu E, Naden R, et al. Identifying Candidate Items Towards the Development of Classification Criteria for Chronic Nonbacterial Osteomyelitis (CNO) and Chronic Recurrent Multifocal Osteomyelitis (CRMO). Ann Rheum Dis 2019;78(Suppl 2):254–5.
93. Bjorksten B, Gustavson KH, Eriksson B, et al. Chronic recurrent multifocal osteomyelitis and pustulosis palmoplantaris. J Pediatr 1978;93:227–31.
94. Jurik AG. Chronic recurrent multifocal osteomyelitis. Semin Musculoskelet Radiol 2004;8:243–53.
95. Schnabel A, Range U, Hahn G, et al. Treatment Response and Longterm Outcomes in Children with Chronic Nonbacterial Osteomyelitis. J Rheumatol 2017;44:1058–65.
96. Eleftheriou D, Gerschman T, Sebire N, et al. Biologic therapy in refractory chronic non-bacterial osteomyelitis of childhood. Rheumatology 2010;49: 1505–12.
97. Zhao Y, Chauvin NA, Jaramillo D, et al. Aggressive therapy reduces disease activity without skeletal damage progression in chronic nonbacterial osteomyelitis. J Rheumatol 2015;42:1245–51.
98. Hospach T, Langendoerfer M, von Kalle T, et al. Spinal involvement in chronic recurrent multifocal osteomyelitis (CRMO) in childhood and effect of pamidronate. Eur J Pediatr 2010;169:1105–11.
99. Zhao Y, Wu EY, Oliver MS, et al. Consensus treatment plans for chronic nonbacterial osteomyelitis refractory to nonsteroidal antiinflammatory drugs and/or with active spinal lesions. Arthritis Care Res 2018;70:1228–37.
100. Padeh S, Brezniak N, Zemer D, et al. Periodic fever, aphthous stomatitis, pharyngitis, and adenopathy syndrome: clinical characteristics and outcome. J Pediatr 1999;135:98–101.
101. Feder HM Jr. Cimetidine treatment for periodic fever associated with aphthous stomatitis, pharyngitis and cervical adenitis. Pediatr Infect Dis J 1992;11: 318–21.
102. Burton MJ, Pollard AJ, Ramsden JD, et al. Tonsillectomy for periodic fever, aphthous stomatitis, pharyngitis and cervical adenitis syndrome (PFAPA). Cochrane Database Syst Rev 2019;(12):CD008669.

Moving?

Make sure your subscription moves with you!

To notify us of your new address, find your **Clinics Account Number** (located on your mailing label above your name), and contact customer service at:

Email: journalscustomerservice-usa@elsevier.com

800-654-2452 (subscribers in the U.S. & Canada)
314-447-8871 (subscribers outside of the U.S. & Canada)

Fax number: 314-447-8029

Elsevier Health Sciences Division
Subscription Customer Service
3251 Riverport Lane
Maryland Heights, MO 63043

*To ensure uninterrupted delivery of your subscription,
please notify us at least 4 weeks in advance of move.